Reiki

for Emotional Healing

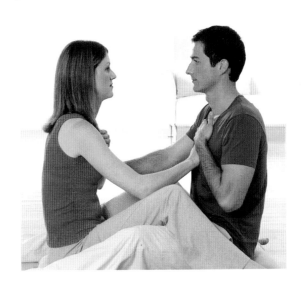

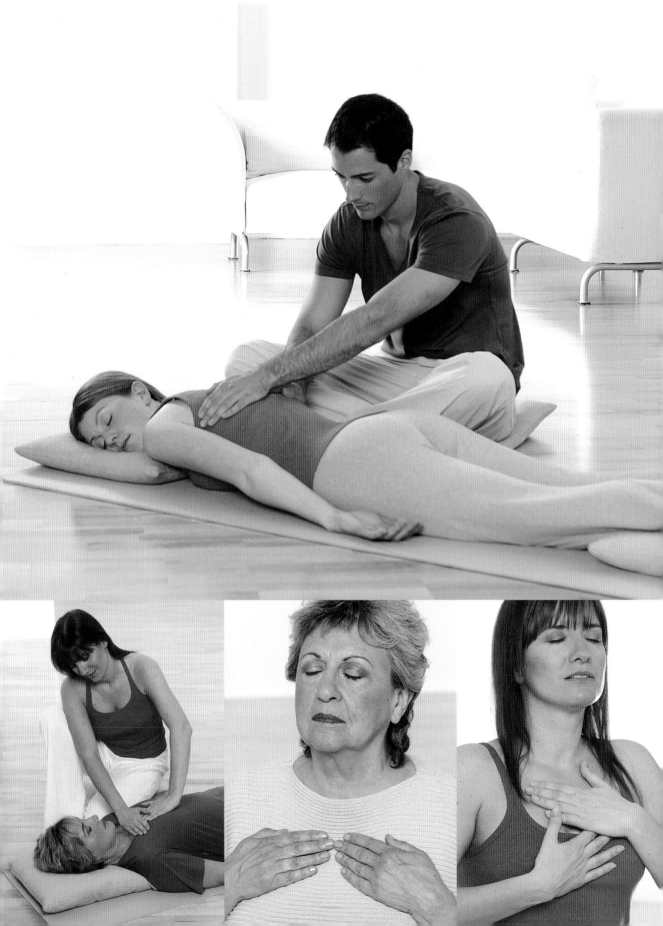

Reiki
for Emotional Healing

TANMAYA HONERVOGT

Reiki Master-Teacher

Gaia Books

Books from Gaia celebrate the vision of Gaia, the self-sustaining living Earth, and seek to help its readers live in greater personal and planetary harmony.

Project Editor Kelly Thompson
Design Hugh Schermuly
Photography Mike Good
Direction Jo Godfrey Wood, Patrick Nugent
Production Simone Nauerth

® This is a Registered Trade Mark of Gaia Books

First published in the United Kingdom in 2006 by:
Gaia Books, an imprint of Octopus Publishing Group Ltd
2–4 Heron Quays, Canary Wharf, London, E14 4JP

Illustrations and compilation © Gaia Books, 2006
Text © Tanmaya Honervogt, 2006

Distributed in the United States and Canada by
Sterling Publishing Co., Inc.
387 Park Avenue South, New York, NY 10016–8810

A CIP catalogue record of this book is available from the British Library:

ISBN-13: 978-1-85675-238-1
ISBN-10: 1-85675-238-0

Printed and bound in China by Toppan
10 9 8 7 6 5 4 3 2 1

Dedication

To all readers of this book and all your friends, loved ones and colleagues:

May your lives unfold with joy, love, peace and happiness, and may this book inspire you to go deeper within, rejoicing in your true self.

Caution

The exercises, hand positions and meditations described in this book are intended for the healing and harmonisation of all living things. The author nevertheless wishes to point out that, in the case of serious illness, a medical doctor should be consulted. The Reiki positions described may naturally be applied as an additional form of treatment. Neither the author nor the publisher accepts any responsibility for the practice or application of the methods described in this book.

About the Author

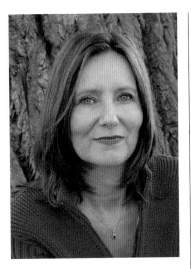

TANMAYA HONERVOGT

TANMAYA HONERVOGT is a Reiki Master-Teacher, author, healer and seminar leader. She spends her time between Germany and England, and travels extensively giving lectures and leading training courses.

Tanmaya is part of the spiritual tradition started by Mikao Usui, the founder of Reiki, and her lineage goes directly back to the source. She trained with one of the few Masters initiated by Hawayo Takata, who introduced Reiki to the Western World in the 1930s.

Tanmaya founded the School of Usui Reiki in 1995 in Devon, England. The school provides a series of certified training courses in the traditional Usui Method. Tanmaya welcomes hearing from Reiki students and readers. She can be contacted via www.tanmaya.info or by writing to: School of Usui Reiki, P.O. Box 2, Chulmleigh, Devon, UK, EX18 7SS.

Prologue

MOST OF THIS BOOK'S CONTENT has developed from the Reiki training courses I have led over the past fifteen years with students from all over the world. Time and time again I have realised how deep a need there is for people to have some kind of help with the emotional and spiritual issues in their lives. After all, we all find ourselves, at times, in awkward or painful situations, where we experience difficult life transitions and emotional problems that we must learn to come to terms with.

In this book I have tried to share my own insights about the challenges we all face in life at times – whether falling ill, losing a loved one, entering the menopause or experiencing a midlife crisis – you name it. The guidance I offer throughout the book is based on my own experiences and learning in my spiritual journey of self-discovery over the last thirty years. I have been fortunate enough to be guided by life to learn about Reiki and meditation; and to be able to meet spiritual teachers and contemporary mystics such as Osho. This has opened a lot of space within me to come closer to who I really am. The longing that we all share to overcome our separation from what we truly are and return to our essence – to rediscover that which has never been lost, where we can deeply relax and experience oneness – is an ongoing adventure that I feel blessed to be part of.

I wish you inspiration in reading and practising what you find in the pages of this book, and hope that you will receive further insights into your life and especially into "who you are" in truth – a divine being having a precious human experience.

Tanmaya Honervogt

Contents

Introduction

Reiki is an ancient hands-on healing technique, rediscovered in ancient Buddhist scriptures at the end of the 19th century by a Japanese monk, Dr Mikao Usui. It is a simple and natural healing method through which we transfer Universal Life Energy for healing from one person to another through the hands.

The word "Rei-ki" (pronounced "ray-key") is a Japanese word literally meaning "Universal Life Energy", which is defined as being the power that acts and lives in all created matter. The syllable "rei" describes the boundless, universal aspect of this energy, while "ki" is the vital energy (or life force) in itself, which flows through all living beings.

Once you become a channel for this energy via the attunement process (see right), you will feel concentrated life energy flowing through your arms and hands of its own accord – an enriching asset that you will retain for the rest of your life. Reiki can be learned by anyone who is open and willing to recognise this healing energy flowing through them.

The Origins of Reiki

Reiki goes back to ancient Buddhist scriptures, in which Mikao Usui found the Reiki symbols and mantras – known as the "formula" – the unique key to the Reiki healing method. Usui undertook a 21-day meditation and fast on sacred Mount Kurama, near Kyoto, in Japan. On the last day of his meditation he found himself in a state of extended consciousness, in which the meaning and use of the symbols were revealed to him. Simultaneously, he felt empowered by the symbols and charged with a powerful

霊
気

healing force. Thus the Usui System of Reiki was born. The full History of Reiki can be read in *Reiki – Healing and harmony through the hands* (see p. 144).

The Attunement Process

To become a "channel" for Universal Life Energy you will receive what is called an "attunement" to the Reiki power. These attunements, during which the Reiki Master transmits energy to the student using an ancient Tibetan technique, are also called "energy transmissions'" or "initiations". The attunement process usually takes the form of a simple ceremony in which the Reiki Master uses the confidential Reiki symbols and mantras. These stimulate and activate the healing channel in the body in order to amplify the flow of energy. The energy enters the body of the student (or recipient) through the top of the head, and flows through the energy centres, called chakras (see p. 140), and down the arms until it leaves the body through the hands. Attunement is the special key to the Reiki system and makes it quite different from any other hands-on healing technique.

The Three Degrees

There are three levels of attunement: First, Second and Third Degree. It is vital to understand that Reiki symbols and mantras are only taught to students of the Second and Third Degrees, which is why we cannot show or explain them in this book. We can say, however, that the First symbol activates the energy available; the Second symbol brings about a sense of harmony and balance and is used especially for mental healing (see p. 24); the Third symbol opens up intuition and is used in distant healing (see p. 139); and the Fourth symbol strengthens the ability to open up to even higher energies and supports meditation. Beginners to Reiki, however, should not be put off, as you can practise all the treatments and exercises in this book without the symbols and mantras. Their effect will simply be stronger if you have undergone official Reiki training.

About this Book

This book aims to guide all levels of Reiki practitioner – from beginner to the most advanced – in using Reiki and other healing techniques to help you meet even the most challenging of situations in a more centred, relaxed and creative way. Reiki can be useful whether you need to make a crucial decision that affects the whole direction of your life or you are merely encountering difficulties at work, within the family or in your relationships. Becoming more in touch with the heart via Reiki will help you to open up and put into action the positive qualities within yourself, such as understanding, compassion and forgiveness. This is because the heart has the capacity to transform any negative energy into its positive opposite.

The Healing Power of the Heart

Most people tend to lose touch with their heart and its healing power. Society and its educational systems focus on training the head, not the heart, and, as a result, most people only know themselves on the surface. Rarely do they come in contact with the true inner depths either of themselves or of others. The first step in reconnecting with the inner wisdom of the heart is to learn to give yourself a little time and energy for silent moments throughout your daily life. Then you will know better what love and peace are.

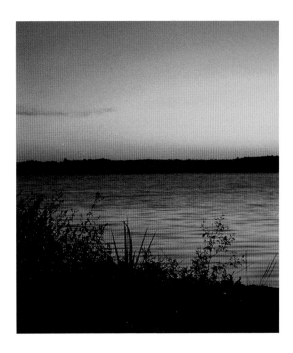

This love and peace come from the very.source of your being. All you need to do to connect with it is to relax your body, mind and emotions. The combination of healing techniques in this book will help you gain more self-knowledge, and the more you understand yourself and value your uniqueness, the easier you will find it to connect with others in a more harmonious way.

Positive Outlook

This book also aims to help you to develop your innate capacity for viewing even apparently difficult situations in a positive way – as stepping stones for inner growth. It encourages you to ask questions, review your values in life and become aware of any limitations you are creating for yourself. In this way, the Reiki techniques are offered as tools for self-exploration, improving your relationships with others and encouraging an expanded sense of well-being that will allow you to live life more fully, with a greater sense of celebration, awareness and contentedness.

The Art of Caring

The book focuses on caring for people of all ages, from babies to the elderly, who are facing a variety of challenges in life. Today there is an ever-increasing need for emotional healing – of the self and of others. And Reiki is a non-intrusive, life-enriching way of offering this – a simple and practical tool to support the healing of physical, mental, emotional and spiritual problems. The book includes a wide variety of self-treatments, as well as treatments for others, as it is vital to recognise that you must first love and heal yourself before you can offer love and healing to others.

Reiki and Meditation

Reiki and meditation are natural partners. You will therefore find a range of valuable meditation and visualisation techniques in this book as well as Reiki treatments, all of which will help you to centre yourself and deepen the connection between body, mind and soul. These exercises relax you, support the healing process and enhance your sense of well-being.

Healing Reactions

It is important to be aware when giving or receiving a Reiki treatment that both physical and emotional "healing reactions" may occur. These are a natural and often necessary part of the healing process, as any "toxic energy" and suppressed emotions held in the body have to rise to the surface before they can be released. For example, on a physical level, a feeling of chilliness during or after a treatment may change after a short time into a pleasant feeling of warmth, a headache may become more intense before getting better or you may feel an urgency to go to the bathroom. On an emotional level, strong emotions from the past may surface. These

"symptoms" can last from ten minutes up to about twenty-four hours. The important thing is just to accept them, let them happen and know that they will soon pass. You will then be one step further down the road to inner harmony.

How To Use the Book

Feel free to use this book in a spontaneous and easy way. You can open it on any page that you feel attracted to explore and use your chosen Reiki treatment or exercises as you wish, as each one can be adapted according to individual needs and knowledge. The chapter titles and sub-sections are there to give you guidance as to which sections may be most appropriate and useful for you.

It is most helpful to use the Reiki treatments and other healing exercises on a daily basis, or at least four to five times during the week. Continue the treatments and exercises for a minimum of three weeks to experience their full effects.

The following ten pages provide you with all the basic Reiki hand positions that make up a full treatment. These positions are slightly different when you do them on yourself to when you do them on another person, which is why we provide you with both a *Full Reiki treatment* to practise on someone else (see pp. 12–17) and a *Self-treatment sequence* (see pp. 18–21). The shorter Reiki treatments throughout this book, recommended to help with specific issues, are actually made up of combinations of these basic hand positions with other variations added in to make the treatments more comprehensive. With practice, however, all sorts of combinations of these hand positions can be used on yourself and others to great effect, so just relax, follow your instincts and enjoy the great healing benefits of Reiki.

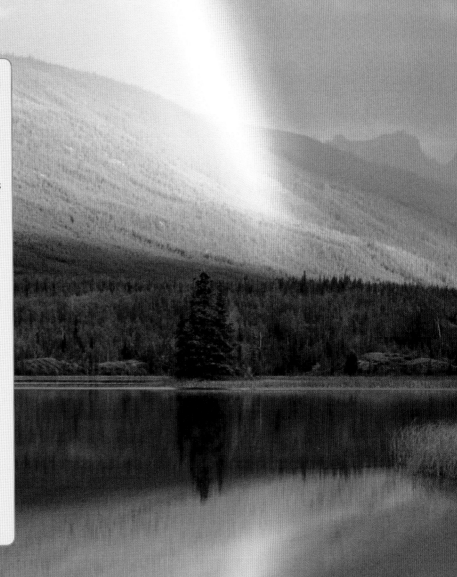

> "There is nothing to do
> other than rest in the power
> that knows the way."
>
> **ROBERT ADAMS,
> CONTEMPORARY MYSTIC**

MAIN REIKI BENEFITS

- *Restores the body's natural energy balance and supports its ability to heal itself.*
- *Promotes deep relaxation, evoking a sense of peace and well-being.*
- *Vitalises both body and soul, thus providing a holistic treatment.*
- *Strengthens the immune system.*
- *Relieves pain and stress.*
- *Helps with many physical ailments, whether they are chronic or acute.*
- *Re-establishes spiritual equilibrium and mental well-being.*
- *Loosens blocked energy and cleanses the body of toxins.*
- *Complements, and can be given in conjunction with, other means of healing, including traditional medical treatment, massage and psychotherapy.*
- *Is non-intrusive, since Reiki energy will pass through all clothing, bandages, plasters, casts and so on.*
- *Is adaptable, according to the need of the recipient.*

Full Reiki treatment

This and the following five pages illustrate the basic Reiki hand positions involved in giving a full-body treatment to another person. It is recommended that you keep your hands in each position for between three and five minutes, which means that you should allow at least an hour to complete it.

It is usual to start a Reiki treatment by first treating the head, then the front of the body, then the back of the body and finally the legs and feet. The person giving the Reiki treatment is known as the "giver" and the person receiving is called the "receiver". It is important that both the giver and receiver are relaxed and comfortable during the treatment as this will maximise the benefits gained. So, while it is important to follow the guidelines given in this book, feel free to adapt the position in which you lie or sit for maximum comfort. It is recommended to wear loose, comfortable clothes that will not cause any restrictions, and to choose a quiet space for the treatment where you will remain undisturbed for the length of the treatment. For treatments best given in a lying position, the receiver can lie on any soft, comfortable surface to which the giver has easy access – a bed, for example, or a couch, a sturdy table with sufficient padding, a mat on the floor or a proper treatment couch.

While giving Reiki, trust your intuition. Sometimes you may sense that a particular area of the receiver's body needs more attention, in which case you can keep your hands there until you feel the energy flow has normalised.

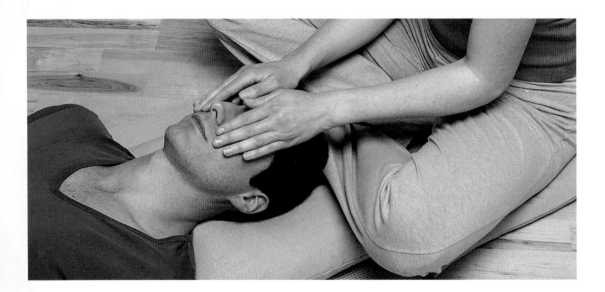

Head Position 1

Place your hands over the receiver's eyes, with your fingers close together. This relaxes the eyes, which in turn relaxes the whole body. It is an ideal way to treat stress or exhaustion.

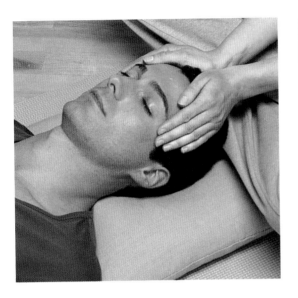

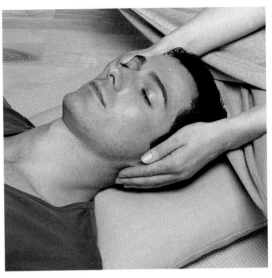

Head Position 2

Place your hands on both sides of the head, above the ears, fingertips touching the temples and palms following the curve of the head. This balances the left and right side of the brain, eases excess mental activity and calms emotions.

Head Position 3

Place your hands over the ears. This allows the receiver to move to a place of deep relaxation within themselves and helps to restore balance to the body. It is particularly good for disorders of the ears and nose, and for colds and flu.

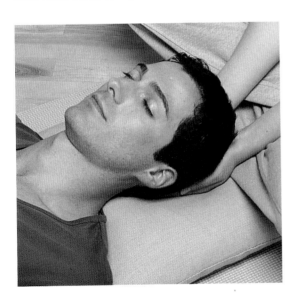

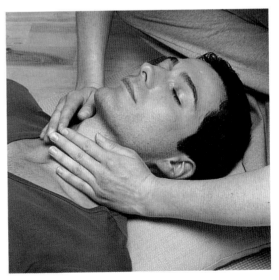

Head Position 4

Cup the back of the head, with the fingertips over the medulla oblongata, an energy point where many nerves connect at the join between the head and the neck. This clarifies thoughts, soothes away tension and calms powerful emotions.

Head Position 5

Place your hands gently above either side of the throat, without directly touching it as it is a very sensitive area. This promotes self-expression, which makes it particularly useful for dealing with suppressed emotions.

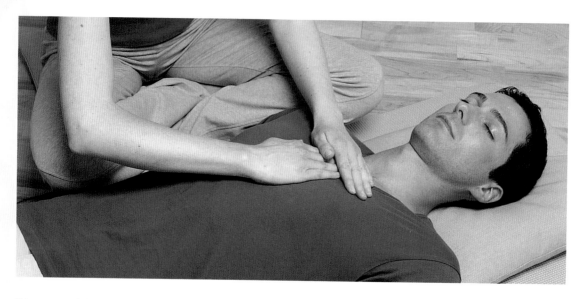

Front Position 1

Place one hand horizontally across the thymus gland, below the collarbone, and the other at right angles to the first in the middle of the chest. This position relates to the heart centre and helps to fortify the immune and lymphatic systems.

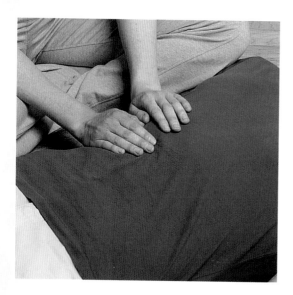

Front Position 2

Place your hands next to each other on the receiver's lower ribs and waist on the right side. This position helps with digestive disorders, aids the detoxification process and balances the emotions.

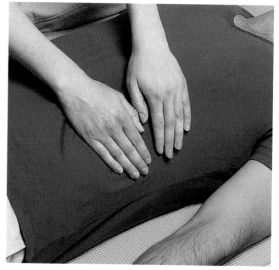

Front Position 3

Place your hands next to each other on the receiver's lower ribs and waist on the left side. This position aids digestion, strengthens the immune system and helps treat infections.

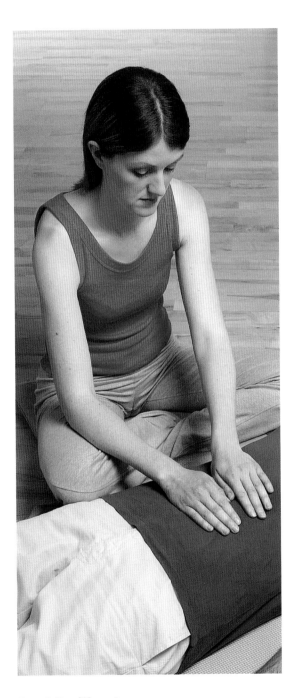

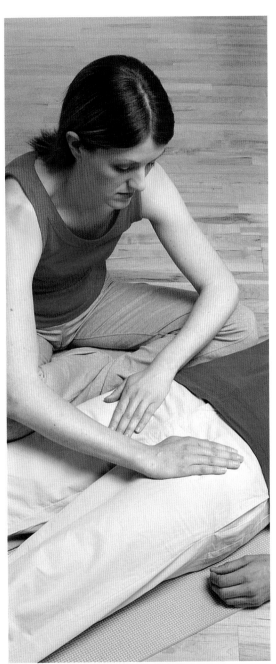

Front Position 4

Place one hand above the navel and the other below it. This
is useful to calm powerful emotions, such as fear, depression
and shock, and helps to restore energy and vitality to the body.
It is also good for indigestion and metabolic disorders.

Front Position 5 (V Position)

Place your hands in a V shape over the pubic area. On a man,
place the hands wide on the groin region. On a woman, place
the hands so that they meet at the point of the V (see p. 20).
This treats the reproductive organs.

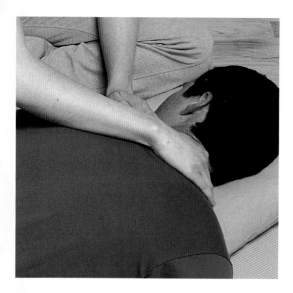

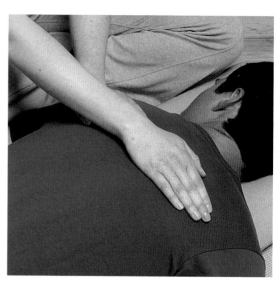

Back Position 1

Place your hands on the receiver's shoulders, one hand to the left and the other to the right of the spine, hands facing in the same direction. This eases tension in the neck and shoulders and helps to release any blocked emotions.

Back Position 2

Place your hands on the shoulder blades, with the fingertips of one hand touching the base of the other palm. This position helps with upper back complaints and promotes the capacity for love, confidence and enjoyment of life.

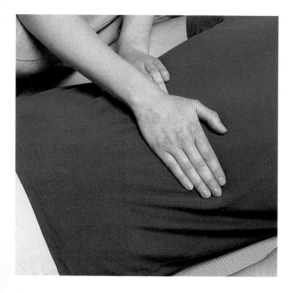

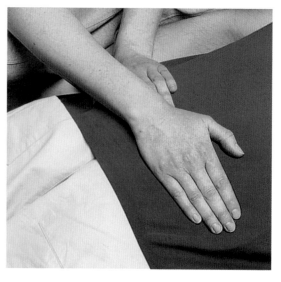

Back Position 3

Place your hands over the lower ribs, over the kidneys. This releases the middle back, helps the body to release toxins and encourages the receiver to let go of any stress and pain from the past.

Back Position 4

If the receiver has a long back, move your hands to the lower part of the back – at hip level – as this eases any lower back pain, strengthens the lymphatic and nervous systems and supports creativity and sexuality.

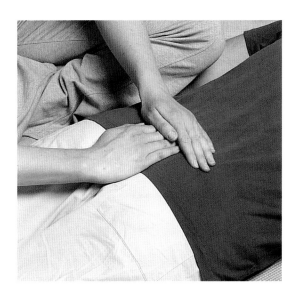

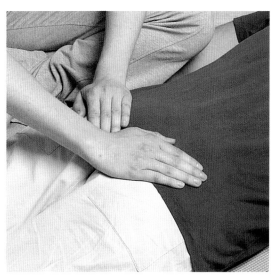

Back Position 5A (T position)

Place one hand across the sacrum and the other at right angles to the first, over the coccyx, to form a T shape. This position helps existential fears and is also useful for haemorrhoids, digestive complaints, bladder disorders and sciatica.

Back Position 5B (V position)

Alternatively, place your hands in a V shape on the receiver's lower back, with the point of the V directly on the coccyx. This position encourages energy to flow more freely up the spine, harmonising the nervous system and promoting confidence.

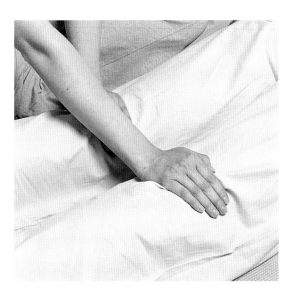

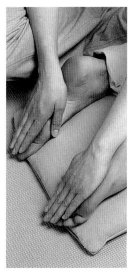

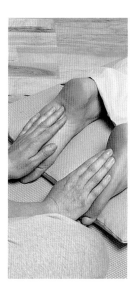

Knee Hollow Position

Cover the back of both knees with your hands. This position is good for treating any knee problems or sport injuries. Emotionally, it also deals with fear, especially the fear of dying.

Sole Positions A or B

Rest your palms on the soles of the receiver's feet. If you cover the toes with your fingertips (A), the receiver may experience a release of energy. If you point your fingers towards the heels (B), the receiver will sense a strong energy flow from feet to head.

Self-treatment sequence

One of the many beautiful aspects of Reiki is that you can treat yourself just as easily as you can treat a friend, colleague or family member. This and the following three pages guide you through the basic hand positions involved in a full self-treatment, starting by treating the head, then moving on to the front of the body and finishing with the back of the body. It is recommended to keep your hands in each position for between three and five minutes, which means you should allow up to an hour to offer yourself the gift of a full Reiki treatment.

Creating the time to do this as often as possible – every day if you can – is likely to have great benefits, making you feel generally calmer, happier and more alert and alive.

Try to choose a time and place where you will be undisturbed for the duration of the treatment so that you can become completely absorbed in what you are doing in the present moment and gain maximum healing benefit from it. Remember to be gentle with yourself by remaining free of any expectations as to what the Reiki "should" do for you. And remember, too, that any symptoms you are experiencing, whether physical or emotional, may become stronger before they balance out and improve, or you may have a strong emotional reaction to the treatment. This is all a natural part of the healing process as the toxins or repressed emotions causing the problems have to come to the surface before they can be released from the body.

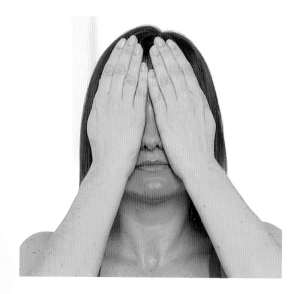

Head Position 1
Place your hands over your eyes, resting your palms on your cheekbones. This position helps to reduce stress, produce clarity of mind and heighten intuition.

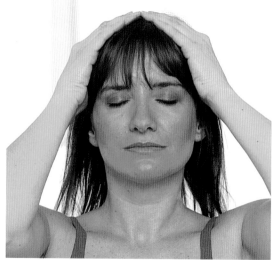

Head Position 2
Place the palm of your hands on your temples, above your ears, and let your fingers follow the curve of your head. This position harmonises the two sides of the brain, improves memory and is helpful for depression and headaches.

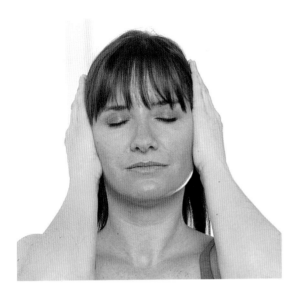

Head Position 3

Place your hands gently over your ears. This position is extremely comforting and is particularly helpful to treat the symptoms of colds, flu or feeling generally run down.

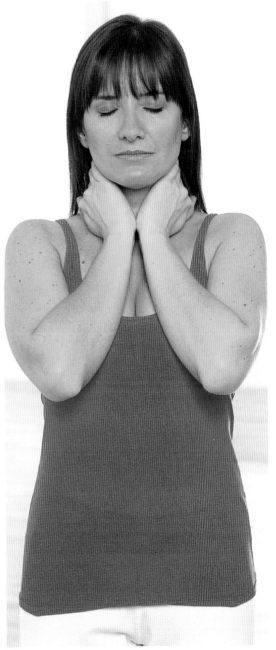

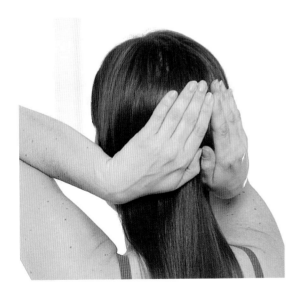

Head Position 4

Cup the back of your head with your hands, fingers pointing upwards. This position promotes a sense of security, relieves fears and depression, calms the mind and emotions, and encourages peaceful sleep.

Head Position 5

Place your hands around your throat, wrists touching at the centre. This harmonises blood pressure and metabolism, helps neck pains and promotes self-expression.

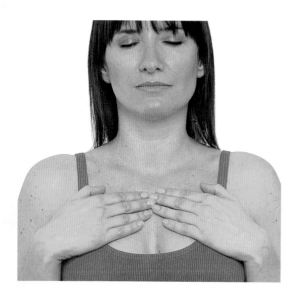

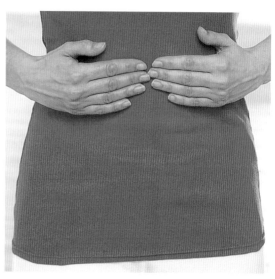

Front Position 1

Place your hands on either side of your chest, fingers touching just below the collarbone. This strengthens the immune system, regulates heart and blood pressure and increases the capacity for love and enjoyment of life.

Front Position 2

Place your hands over the lower ribcage, above the waist, fingers touching in the middle. This position regulates digestion, increases energy levels, promotes relaxation and reduces fears and frustrations.

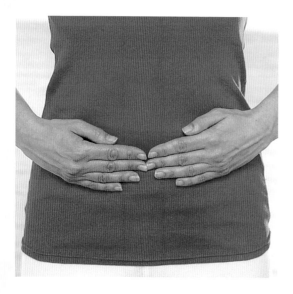

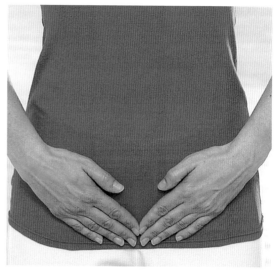

Front Position 3

Place your hands on either side of your navel, fingers touching in the middle. This position regulates metabolism, helps with digestion, eases powerful emotions, such as fear and depression, and boosts your self-confidence.

Front Position 4

Place your hands in a downward-pointing V shape over the pubic area. For women, the fingertips should touch, while for men, the hands should rest wider on the groin area (see p. 15). This treats the sexual organs and gives a sense of grounding.

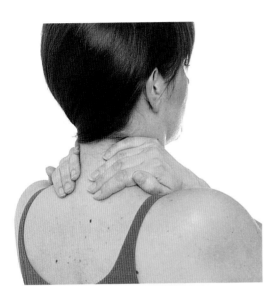

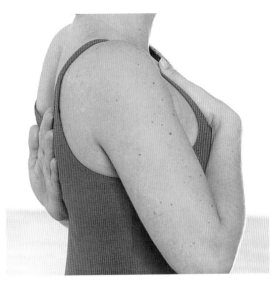

Back Position 1

Place your hands on the upper shoulders, on either side of the spine. This position promotes relaxation and is helpful for shoulder tension, and upper back and neck pain. It also helps to release suppressed emotions.

Back Position 2

Place one hand in the middle of the chest and the other at the same height on your back, palm facing outward. This position balances the thymus gland, harmonises the heart, stimulates the immune system and increases confidence.

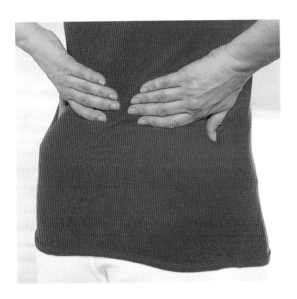

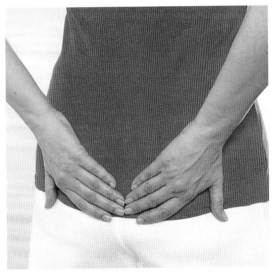

Back Position 3

Place your hands around your waist, at kidney-height, fingers pointing towards the spine. This position strengthens the kidneys, adrenal glands and nerves, promotes detoxification, eases back pain and reinforces self-esteem.

Back Position 4

Place your hands in a downward-pointing V shape so that your fingers touch your coccyx. This position treats the sexual organs, aids digestion, promotes creativity and provides a sense of grounding.

Chapter 1

The Relationship with Yourself

"The self is a sea, boundless and measureless. Say not, 'I have found the truth,' but rather, 'I have found a truth.' Say not, 'I have found the path of the soul.' Say rather, 'I have met the soul walking upon my path.' … The soul unfolds itself, like a lotus of countless petals."

KAHLIL GIBRAN, *THE PROPHET*, 1923

WE ARE BORN INTO THIS WORLD as complete beings, without preconceptions and expectations, yet already endowed with the Universal Life Force – an energy that sustains us through life and whose levels we can modify for our health and well-being. We have no preconceptions of how things should be, no fixed opinions, no judgements. Instead, we have an openness and a willingness to explore and learn about the world around us.

It doesn't take long, though, before our innocence, natural inquisitiveness and positive relationship with ourselves are diluted by the "rules" of the society in which we are raised. Our innate intelligence means that we learn to control our behaviour and to please others in order to survive. In the process we internalise all kinds of ideals and beliefs that have nothing to do with who we really are. In this way we create a reality that is at odds with our inner being, although this is done unconsciously. Children are often told what is "wrong" with them and are therefore unintentionally "programmed" by those around them to believe that these "faults" are theirs for life. The people who shape our early lives – be they teachers, parents, other relatives or peers – have a powerful impact on how we view ourselves and what we believe about ourselves.

By the time we reach our teens, we are often deeply conditioned in our own behaviour, values and attitudes towards life, thus we have created our own belief systems. These extend well into adult life, creating unnecessary self-restrictions, which can manifest themselves as anything from low self-esteem or patterns of negative behaviour to a generally unhealthy relationship with the self: we try to make the life that we are expected to live work for us, and we invest a lot in personal achievement. Just as we wanted to be a good child, we now want to be a good student, husband, wife, father, mother, employee. And this puts a lot of pressure on us, which burdens us and makes it hard for us to enjoy life fully. It's no wonder we can end up feeling unimportant and unhappy, given that we feel pressure to fulfil so many requirements before we think we are worthy of simply being loved for ourselves.

A lot of time and healing is needed to resolve the inner conflicts that this societal conditioning has caused, and Reiki is an ideal means of doing this. This is because it

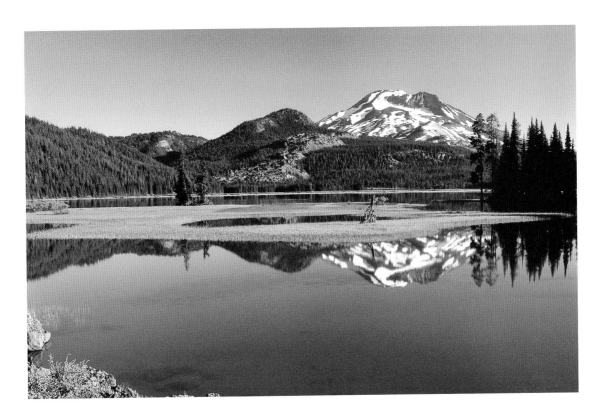

addresses not only the physical but also the mental and emotional levels of our being by tapping into the subtle layer of energy that we call the "emotional body". Reiki treatments – whether on yourself or given by someone else – help us to become aware of any hidden, negative belief systems and encourage us to transform negative patterns by reconnecting us to the Universal Life Force with which we were born, reminding us that life is not a problem to be solved, but a mystery to be lived.

The treatments in this chapter are designed to support us in finding the courage and trust to reveal, and thus start to heal, our worries, insecurities and wounds. The awareness we develop through the treatments encourage us to question our own boundaries, limitations, and deep-seated beliefs that we are unworthy, weak, unattractive, untrustworthy, unintelligent or whatever other qualities we have projected onto ourselves. A sense of humour is

useful when doing this as we all too often play out self-constructed dramas where we – whether knowingly or not – take on the role of the judge or victim.

If we can open our hearts through Reiki and learn to listen to what it wants to tell us, we will discover that the heart is always guiding us to a place of inner peace and contentment.

This chapter is divided into six main sections, all of which are integral when trying to develop a healthier relationship with ourselves: *Becoming aware of belief systems* (see pp. 24–5), *Developing self-love* (see pp. 26–9), *Learning to trust* (see pp. 30–1), *Practising forgiveness* (see pp. 32–3), *Connecting with joy* (see pp. 34–5) and *Self-recognition* (see pp. 36–7). Feel free to work through them in the order they appear or, alternatively, you may wish to dip in and out of whichever section seems most relevant to you at any given time.

Becoming aware of belief systems

FROM THE MOMENT WE ARE BORN society and the people around us unknowingly "programme" us. We are given a name, learn that we have an identity – whether boy or girl, Christian or Hindu, American or Japanese – and quickly learn how to behave to fit into this notion of who we are supposed to be.

At the age of about two and a half, we start to become aware of our own identity as a separate being, gain a sense of "I" and "me", and say "no" to certain things, thus already forming our own beliefs and judgements. At the same time, however, we are very impressionable, which means it is easy for us to feel that we "fall short" of people's expectations when we are told off or put down. The force of the unconscious mind is powerful, so negative beliefs about ourselves all too easily travel with us into adult life.

As long as we are not aware of the conditioning, life will always be the way we believe it must be. By clinging to our ingrained negative beliefs, we will always unconsciously create circumstances in life that reinforce the negative patterns of our childhood. On the other hand, if we become aware of the belief systems we carry, we can allow ourselves to see their limitations and finally let go of them, thus taking the first step on the road to emotional well-being. Reiki can help us access and transform these deeply seated beliefs and judgements about ourselves by bringing them to the conscious mind.

Reiki Mental Healing: Self-treatment

This healing technique – which is usually taught in the Second Degree, but is offered here for all levels, with a more advanced option – allows you to ask the unconscious and super-conscious mind, or the "Higher Self", for guidance in bringing healing via the spirit. Allow about ten to fifteen minutes for the whole process.

If you are attuned to **Reiki Second Degree**, *you can use the symbols taught by your Reiki teacher before placing your hands in Step 2. Draw the Second Reiki symbol and then the First symbol on the back of the head, while saying the corresponding mantras and your own name three times.*

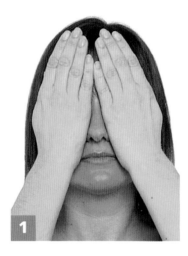

1 Sit on a chair with both feet on the floor, or lie on your back, and cover your eyes with your palms for a few moments. Second Degree practitioners, see box left.

2 Place your right hand over the crown chakra (see p. 140) on the top of your head with your fingertips pointing

backwards; and place your left hand on the back of your head with the palm covering the medulla oblongata, where the head joins the neck. Then close your eyes and visualise a beam of loving light entering your body through your hands for up to a few minutes.

3 Silently say: *"Make me aware of the cause of my (mention your problem) and show me what I need to do to love, accept and heal myself completely."* Repeat this three times in total and imagine it entering the body through the top of your head. Become aware of any sensations that this causes in your body, or any memories or images that it brings up from your unconscious mind.

4 Once again send love and light into your body via your hands before slowly removing them from your head. Then rub your hands together to break the connection.

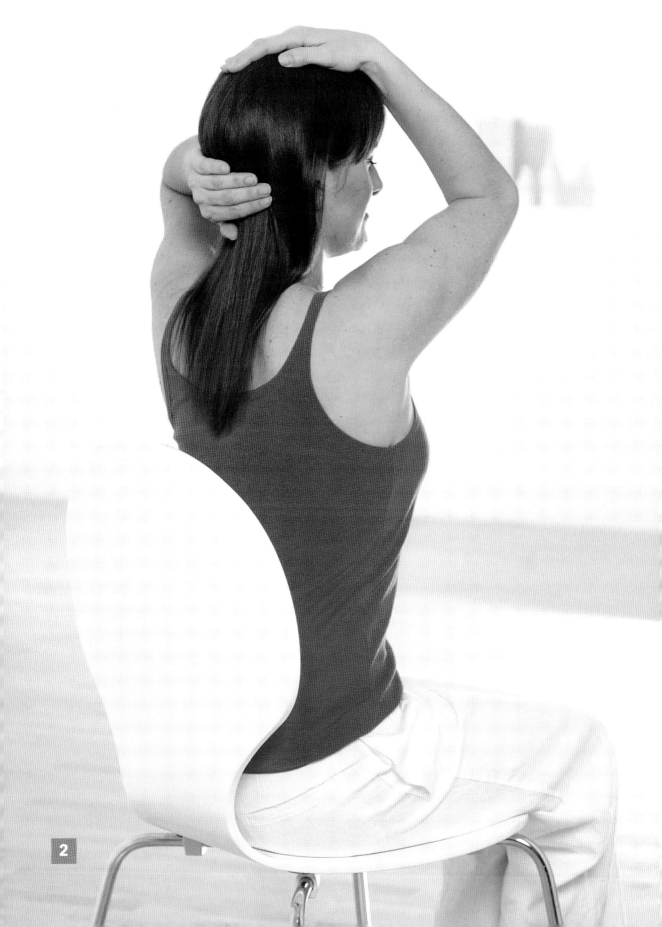

Developing self-love

WE HAVE ALL HEARD the expression "love heals". However, it's really only unconditional love that heals. Much of what we often call love comes with conditions: we love someone because we don't want to be alone, or we think we can get something we need from them. We expect this person to make us happy, and they expect us to make them happy – ironically, the cause of many unhappy relationships. In order to be able to love unconditionally we first have to focus on our relationship with ourselves by learning to accept, respect and unconditionally love ourselves – be our own best friend.

The first step towards this goal is looking at what you believe about yourself (see *Becoming aware of belief systems*, pp. 24–5). If you believe you are not good enough then you cannot look objectively; instead, you judge yourself and expect yourself to be perfect. It is time to pull down the walls of your own limitations and negative beliefs. Forgive yourself for not being "perfect" and for not loving yourself in the past and start afresh now.

You can only be the way you are. Open your heart and you will once again be able to experience this love and feel the enormous emotional freedom that it brings to you. When you discover this source of love within yourself, you can finally accept who you are and accept others the way they are, as you cannot really love others until you love yourself.

Listening to the Heart: Exercise

The key to reconnecting with yourself and learning to love yourself again lies in the heart – the seat of all love and compassion. This exercise will help you to become more in touch with your innermost feelings. Allow between ten and fifteen minutes to do it.

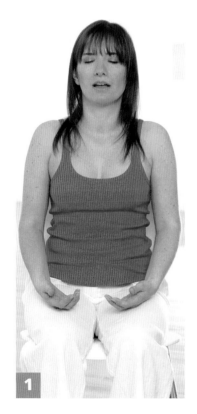

1 Sit or lie down, take a few deep, relaxing breaths and, if you sense tension in the body or heaviness in the heart, try sighing to gain relief.

2 Place both hands on your heart, connect with your heart chakra and feel your heartbeat for a few minutes. Continue to sigh, releasing any pressure from the heart with each sigh.

3 Now start talking to your heart, as if it were an old friend. You can ask questions, such as, *"How are you?"* and *"Can I do something for you?"* Allow any feelings that come up to just be there – there's no need to do anything with them.

Connecting with Inner Peace: Exercise

This exercise is a perfect way either to start or end your day. However, you can also do it at times when you are feeling ill at ease with yourself for some reason, as the low humming sound harmonises the heart centre and brings you in contact with the love and peace that emanates from here.

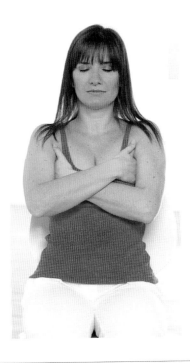

1 Sit with your eyes closed and your hands resting in your lap or on your upper legs. Breathe naturally and make a deep humming sound on each out-breath for about five minutes, keeping the same note all the way through.

2 Then place your left hand under your right armpit and your right hand under your left armpit, with the thumbs out. You can continue to hum while you do this if you like but it is not necessary. Focus your attention on the chest area and allow your heart to become calm and a feeling of love and peace to arise. Enjoy this feeling for about ten minutes.

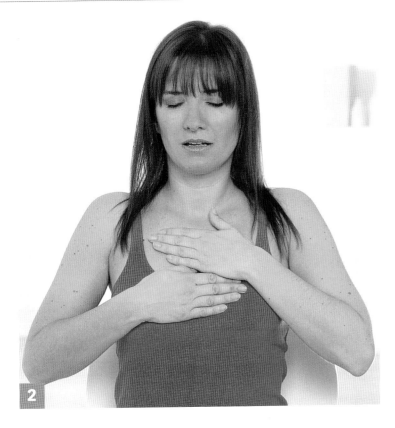

4 After a few moments, say – either silently or out loud – *"I have patience, love and understanding for myself".* Repeat this a few times and notice if it makes you feel more accepting and loving of yourself

Sending Healing Affirmations

Remembering and consciously acknowledging your natural inner resources strengthens your love for yourself, which can, in turn, help to resolve emotional conflicts. This exercise combines the Reiki Mental Healing technique (see pp. 24–5) with the use of healing affirmations in order to do this.

1 Choose one or two positive affirmations that apply to you. You can use one of the examples given (see box, bottom right) or create your own.

2 Sit or lie comfortably on your back, close your eyes and take a few deep breaths, letting go of any tension in the body as you breathe out. Then place your hands over your eyes for a short while, resting your palms on your cheekbones. Relaxing the eyes relaxes the whole body. Second Degree practitioners, see box right.

3 Place your left hand on the back of your head, your palm covering the medulla oblongata, and place your right hand on the top of your crown chakra (see p. 140), fingertips pointing backwards. Keep your hands in this soothing position for the full length of the treatment.

4 Visualise a beam of light entering your body through your palms. Allow your whole body to fill from head to toe with this light, love and energy for two to three minutes.

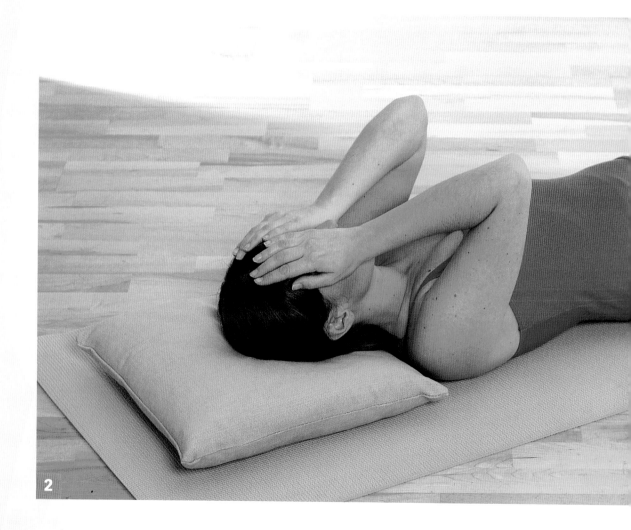

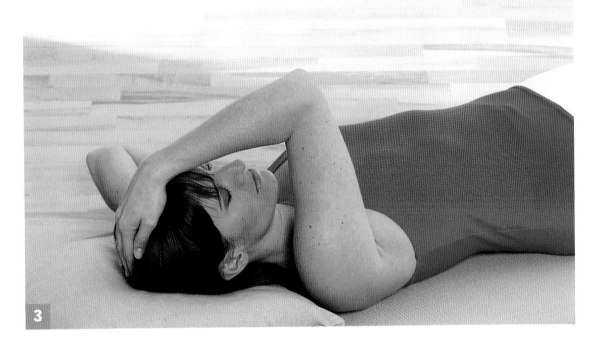

3

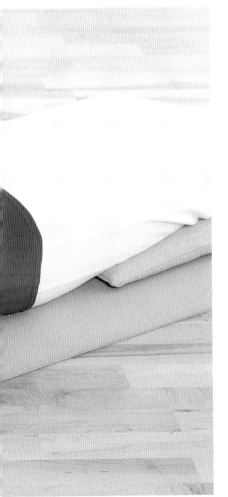

5 Now silently utter your chosen affirmation three times, directing it into your body through the top of the head. Remain fully aware of how you feel as you are doing this and just allow any emotions to arise as they will.

6 Again send light and love into the body through your hands before slowly removing them from your head. Stretch your body gently before coming back to your normal state of awareness.

Second Degree practitioners *can use the Mental Healing symbols by drawing them over the back of your head, before placing your hands in Step 3. Alternatively, visualise the symbols on the back of the head. In both cases, say the mantras of each symbol three times. Rub your hands together after the healing to disconnect from the symbols.*

Healing Affirmations

Healing affirmations help you to reconnect with the positive qualities that already dwell inside you. It is a good idea to work with one affirmation for seven days and then change to another one – you can choose from the list below or create your own.

I accept and love myself the way I am, simply because I am as I am.
I am important and value myself.
I am willing to forgive myself.
I am perfect just the way I am.
I claim and accept my power.
I deserve to be loved.
I deserve the best in life.
I release the need to be perfect.
I am open to receive love and give love.
I am grateful for everything I have and receive in life.
I care about the child in me and know that it is deeply loved by me.

Learning to trust

TRUST DEVELOPS OUT OF LOVE. When you trust yourself you love yourself, and when you love yourself you can trust yourself. It is not the same as "faith", where you have to believe in something or someone else – rather, it is your own experience, your own growth, which brings you to trust. As children, trust came to us naturally, but most people lose this ability as life goes on. If we want to live an emotionally fulfilled life, however, there is a deep need to rediscover this trust, as nobody can truly live happily in a climate of fear and mistrust.

The demands of modern society usually keep us caught up in our heads for most of the time. The head can be useful for solving logical problems, but when it comes to feelings – the things that give us real joy in life – we need to move down from the head and connect with the energy of the heart.

The heart (or heart chakra; see p. 140) is the centre of our soul. It is true and sincere, represents love and acceptance, and when you are centred, you can trust both life and yourself. Relaxation and emotional healing always come from this "heart space".

Reiki can support a shift in our energy focus from the head to the heart. In this way we can reconnect with the heart's natural capacity to enjoy life, to express loving feelings, to trust, and to bring emotional harmony to our actions and feelings.

From Head to Heart: Self-treatment

This treatment strengthens your heart, stimulates your immune system and increases your capacity for love, trust and enjoyment. It can transform feelings of weakness, fear, frustration or depression into ones of joy and happiness. Treating the heart chakra (see pp. 134–5) will bring compassion, while treating the sacral chakra – the second chakra – will bring you more in touch with your innermost desires and increase your self-confidence.

1 Sit or lie down comfortably on your back, close your eyes, and take a few deep, relaxing breaths in and out.

2 Place your hands on the middle of the chest, where your heart chakra is located. Breathe in and expand your lungs with each in-breath, imagining that the air is made of love. Exhale when your lungs are filled with this love. Continue this for about five minutes, before allowing the energy that has gathered in the heart area to sink deeper inside the body.

3 Now move your hands to the abdomen, on either side of the navel. Imagine the air flowing from the chest into the abdomen with each out-breath and relax into the belly area. Stay here for about five minutes.

4 Place one hand below the navel and the other hand on the middle of the chest, on your heart chakra. This connects and balances the energy between the belly (sacral chakra) and the heart (heart chakra). Again, stay in this position for about five minutes.

"Reiki has become my place of refuge. My body and mind relax with Reiki and my worries and fears dissolve."

SUSIE, 34, REIKI STUDENT

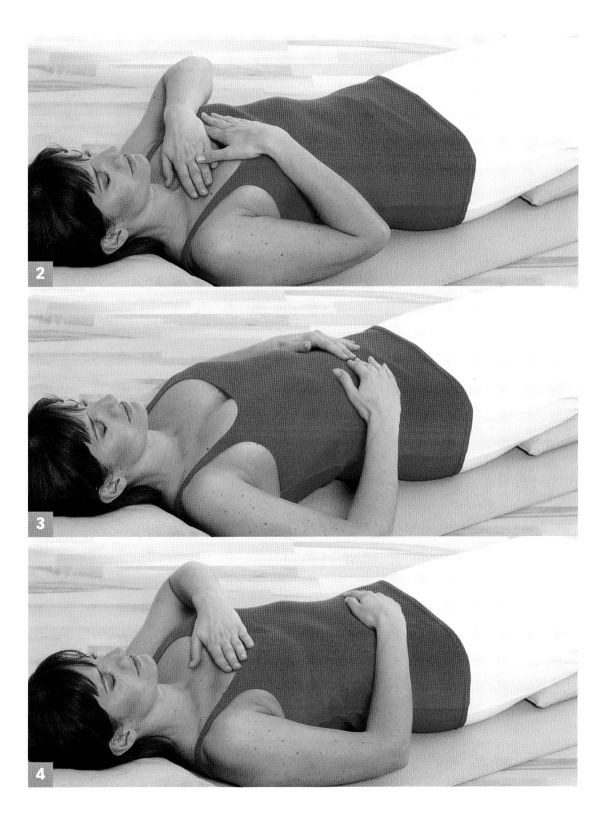

Practising forgiveness

BUDDHIST TEACHINGS say that, in truth, everything and everyone is interconnected and interdependent. Thus everything we do to others is actually being done to ourselves: the principle of cause and effect called karma. When we are unaware of this interconnectedness and the consequences of our harmful actions, we can hurt each other carelessly, without awareness of what we are doing.

So, when you find yourself holding grudges against others, turn inwards and take an honest look at your own motivations and actions. Once you recognise your own weaknesses and faults – which have inevitably hurt others from time to time, albeit unintentionally – how can you possibly feel angry and resentful towards another person?

Forgiving ourselves and forgiving other people therefore become one and the same thing. We need to forgive others because we do not want to suffer any more each time we remember what they did – or how we reacted. When we feel bad about something we did, we sub-consciously punish ourselves by feeling guilty, ashamed or worthless, which, in turn, makes us feel ill at ease and unable to relax. Ultimately, forgiving shows compassion for ourselves and a desire to let old wounds heal, rather than fester. So start now: forgive yourself – and everyone around you – for everything in the past. Forgiveness brings us back in touch with our heart, healing our emotions and clearing out all the emotional baggage weighing us down.

Forgiving Yourself: Meditation

This meditation helps you to recognise and let go of past feelings of guilt and blame that you have been hanging on to, thus opening the doors to increased emotional freedom, lightness and acceptance.

1 Sit comfortably with your eyes closed and take a few deep, relaxing breaths. Place one or both hands around the navel, noticing the rise and fall of your belly while you are breathing. Try to relax even more deeply into this area of your body.

2 Think of a situation for which you want to forgive yourself. For example, you can forgive yourself for criticising yourself, for the wounds and dramas you have created in your life or for not loving or supporting yourself enough.

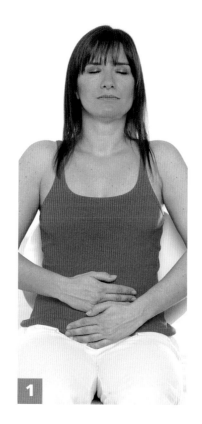

1

3 Shift your hands from the belly to the heart centre in the middle of the chest, and feel the connection with your heart. Now say to yourself:
" I forgive myself for (fill in your own words)…"
Say the sentence three times out loud so that you can hear it clearly. Saying it might conjure up strong memories or images of the situation upon which you are working, so if emotions come up, just allow them to happen. There's no need to do anything else with them. Feel compassion for yourself, and if more situations appear that you would like to forgive yourself for, simply repeat the process with a new, relevant sentence.

4 After the exercise take a few moments to rest and then come back to normal consciousness.

"When even my dearest friend, whom I had helped,

Unexpectedly turns against me,

May I view him as a great treasure, difficult to find."

GESHE LANGRI THANGPA, TIBETAN BUDDHIST

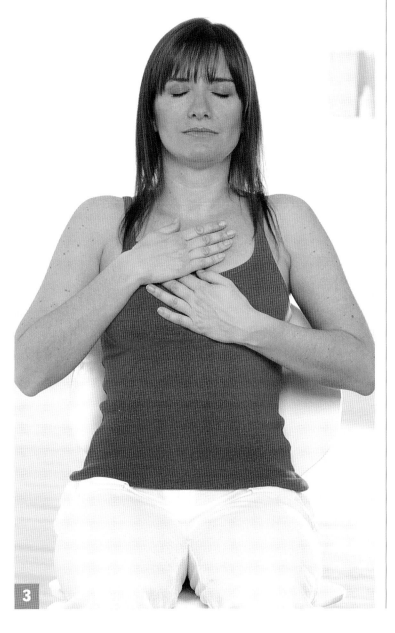

3

Forgiving Another Person

It is just as important to forgive other people as it is to forgive yourself, as nothing is resolved by holding on to anger and resentment. Whatever they did is likely to have little to do with you and much more to do with their own world of drama, confusion and reactions – a mirror of their old, unacknowledged wounds. In knowing this, we can stop taking things so personally, which allows us to feel more compassion and have more understanding for ourselves and others.

When we release the hurt that we have carried inside us, we open up to a life of compassion and understanding, rather than guilt, blame and shame. And we may even find that a person who has appeared to be our enemy has, in fact, enriched our life, helping us to soften our hearts.

Use the same technique as for *Forgiving Yourself* (see left) to forgive another person, only this time use a sentence that involves someone else who you want to forgive, for example, "I want to forgive my mother for not having enough time for me when I was little." As before, make sure you take adequate rest at the end of the session.

Connecting with joy

JOY IS A QUALITY OF THE HEART that happens when your body, mind and heart all function in harmony. Joy contains something of pleasure, of happiness, and yet it is somehow more – like when children sometimes laugh for no apparent reason. When you are joyful your body is relaxed, your mind is calm and your heart is overflowing with energy, love and peace. The key to finding such joy is connecting on a deep level with your heart, as the heart naturally knows how to relax, enjoy and celebrate life. Giving Reiki to the heart opens it up and helps the healing energy flow to this area.

Atisha – an ancient Tibetan Master who developed the meditation below – discovered that we can absorb anything that has been causing suffering into the empty space of our heart. Fear, worry, anxiety, struggle, feelings of unworthiness, judgements and so on – all these "ghosts" are welcome. As they enter the heart chakra when we breathe in, they dissolve and disappear into the empty space inside the heart. And once the heart absorbs and transforms these negative energies, we can breathe out positive energies, sending them back into the body-mind-heart mechanism.

Atisha's Heart of Joy: Meditation

This meditation is based on the understanding that the deeper we melt into the heart, or the heart chakra, the more we can disappear as a separate "I". The combination of Reiki with this meditation technique deepens the healing experience.

1 Sit relaxed with your eyes closed. Breathe deeply a few times and sigh on each out-breath.

2 Place your hands on the middle of the chest (your heart chakra; see p. 140) and bring to mind a past or current situation that has caused or is causing you pain or suffering. Breathe in and welcome the feeling. If tears come, just let them happen. Accept any emotion that arises and allow yourself to move deeply into the simple energy of the feeling, without the mind putting labels or judgements on it.

3 Then, as you breathe out, reconnect with a feeling of peace, love or joy. Allow the out-breath to carry the blessings of peace, joy and love.

"Keep on knocking til the joy inside

opens a window to see who's there."

RUMI, *SECRET LANGUAGE*, TR. COLEMAN BARKS

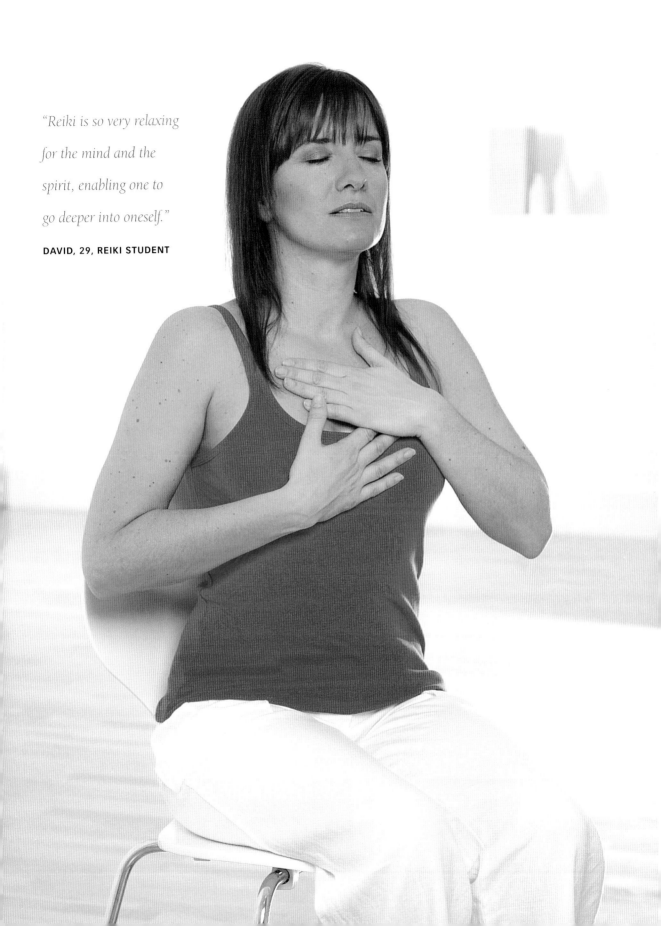

"Reiki is so very relaxing for the mind and the spirit, enabling one to go deeper into oneself."

DAVID, 29, REIKI STUDENT

Self-recognition

WE ALL ARE LOOKING FOR HAPPINESS in life. We think we will be happy when we get what we want, but this is an illusion that keeps us from experiencing the happiness that is available to us here and now. It is the mind that is wanting, the mind that is setting up goals and expectations. But the mind is not the "real" you; it is just a collection of opinions and beliefs that you have gathered in the past. All your expectations are leading you away from yourself, and towards frustration.

You think you are the body, the mind and the emotions but in reality, you are much more. You are a divine being of light and there is silence, peace and unconditional love inside you. You are already perfect the way you are. All you need to do is recognise this and be willing to discover who you really are: look deep inside for the true self that dwells at the still and silent centre, distant from all external events in your life.

Recognising and surrendering to your own nature will mean you have no more resistance to what life brings you, nor suffering because you want it to be different from what it is. Everything will be perfect the way it is. You will be perfect the way you are. And you will be able to let go of all the beliefs and judgements that have made you unhappy in the past. Allow Reiki to lead you down this path of recognition so that the struggling can stop and you can start simply to enjoy life for what it is.

Connecting to the Divine: Exercise

This exercise will help you to open and strengthen the connection to a divine force inside yourself – a "Higher Self" or "spiritual guide" – so that you are no longer an obstacle for your own love, happiness and healing. Suggested treatment time is between fifteen and twenty minutes.

If you are attuned to **Second Degree Reiki** *you can use the Reiki symbols for Mental Healing by drawing the symbols over the back of the head, before placing your hands in Step 2. Alternatively, you can visualise the symbols. In both cases, say the mantras belonging to each symbol three times. Rub your hands at the end of the healing to break the spiritual connection.*

1 Lie down on your back and close your eyes. Take a few deep, relaxing breaths and let go of any thoughts and tensions in the body as you breathe out. Now place your hands over your eyes. Stay here for about five minutes to balance the hormones, reduce emotional stress and facilitate meditation. Second Degree Practitioners, see box left.

2 Then place your right hand on the back of your head, palm covering the medulla oblongata, and your left hand on your crown chakra (see p. 140), fingertips pointing backwards. Keep your hands here for about ten minutes.

3 Visualise a beam of light entering your body through your palms and let your whole body fill with this love and energy for a few minutes. Send extra light to any darker areas of the body that you might find.

4 Imagine that the door to the room you are in has opened and a higher force than you – a divine energy – is entering. Gently ask this force to offer you healing. Ask it questions about yourself if you like, such as *"What is the next step in my life?"* and wait for answers to arise. Allow about ten minutes for this, before thanking the higher force.

5 Then visualise more light, love and healing entering your body through your hands before slowly removing them from your head. Stretch your body gently to help you come back to your normal state of consciousness.

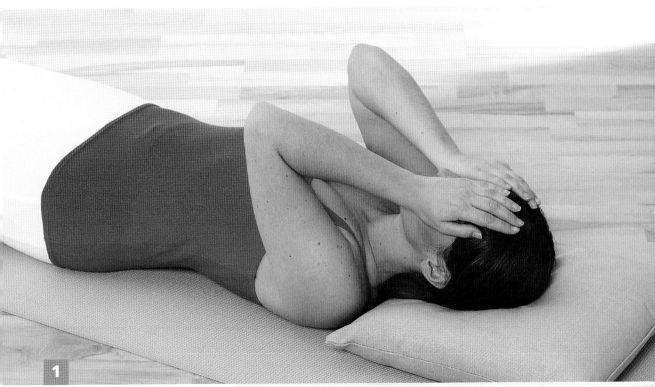

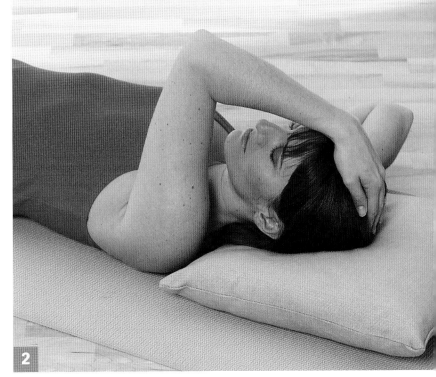

"Reiki has turned my life around. I have found real contentment and enjoyment through practising Reiki everyday on myself, my family and my friends. I am learning all the time about myself and building my confidence."

THOMAS, 24, REIKI STUDENT

Chapter 2
Home Life

"It is well to give when asked, but it is better to give unasked, through understanding; and to the open-handed the search for one who shall receive is joy greater than giving, and is there aught you would withhold? All you have shall some day be given; therefore give now, that the season of giving may be yours and not your inheritors."

KAHLIL GIBRAN, *THE PROPHET,* **1923**

OUR WAYS OF LIVING change throughout life: first we live with our parents; then we leave home and live on our own or with a partner; and eventually we may become parents and start the whole cycle again by having children of our own. However, people live together in all sorts of scenarios these days: whether with same-sex partners, as single parents with children, as new families with step-children from previous relationships or together with friends or like-minded people.

We all know from experience that living with others can bring up conflict and problems. We can easily find ourselves in what we view as complicated, unhappy situations. Despite our longing to have loving relationships with those around us, other people often end up "getting on our nerves", as they don't behave in the way we want or expect them to. However, by projecting outside of ourselves and blaming others for certain things – as we all too often do – we set a trap for ourselves. The fact that, in our minds, it is "their fault" that things are not going right and that we are not responsible makes us the victims, with no way out. We have given away our power and, with it, any possibility to change the situation.

This can have a far-reaching effect on our lives, as the peaceful and harmonious home setting to which most of us aspire dissolves before our eyes, and our need and desire to have a place of sanctuary from the hectic world around us remain unfulfilled. Thankfully, then, there are lots of ways to improve unhealthy relationships at home and even to make good living circumstances and relationships better still.

Making an effort to become more aware of all the aspects of your own personality – from beliefs and opinions, judgements and habits, to likes and dislikes – is a good place to start. Reiki allows you to deepen this self-awareness, which often removes many of the obstacles to harmonious relationships with the people around you. By tapping into the Universal Life Energy we are able to expand and raise our level of consciousness, as well as balance strong emotions and bring harmony to the body's system and clarity to the mind.

This chapter is all about getting the very best from the time we spend at home. It is divided into eight sections as a guide to help you to choose which exercises are most relevant to you and your life. The first four sections –

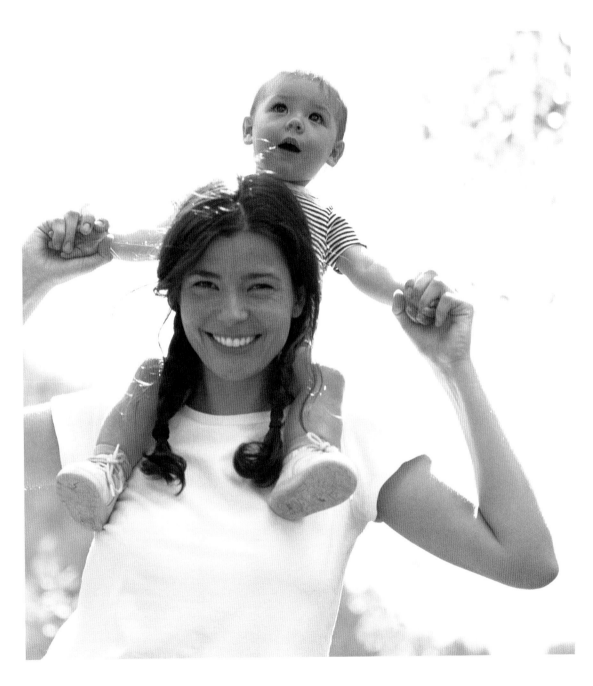

Relating to others (see pp. 40–1), *Supporting intimacy* (see pp. 42–5), *Sharing* (see pp. 46–7) and *Accepting* (see pp. 48–51) – help you to become more aware of how your own behaviour affects the relationships with the people you live with. The latter four sections of the chapter –

Treating children (see pp. 52–5), *Treating babies* (see pp. 56–7), *Treating older people* (see pp. 58–9) and *Treating pets & plants* (see pp. 60–61) – encourage you to offer Reiki as a gift to those with whom you live and about whom you care.

Relating to others

THE WAY YOU RELATE TO THE OTHER PEOPLE you live with is key to how happy a home life you have, and how strong your unique bond with each person is.

It is useful to try to view all your relationships with other people as a mirror. If you can honestly and objectively examine the behaviour of a person who upsets you or makes you angry, you will find that anything that particularly disturbs you is often reflecting some part of yourself that you don't like and/or have not acknowledged. Whatever you dislike in the other person you will usually find hidden somewhere in yourself. It is important to know and own this part of your own self, so that you can love and accept yourself as a whole human being – and thus accept others in the same way. Whenever you find a judgement arising about another, try the exercise below.

As long as we are not aware of our wounds, it is likely that we will keep attracting situations and people who stir up the same hurtful feelings that we have experienced in the past. For healing to happen the hurt needs to be exposed, otherwise it will keep festering and waiting for the next opportunity to get our attention.

Reiki helps to prepare the ground for the healing process to happen as it balances strong emotions, brings harmony to the body's systems and increases clarity of mind, all of which allow you to relate in a more harmonious ways to others.

Insights into Projection

To become aware of the judgements you make on others, find a quiet space where nobody will disturb you for the fifteen to thirty minutes this exercise takes to complete. You will need a pen and paper or your journal nearby.

1 Sit down, take a few deep breaths and bring to mind a situation where you felt sad, disturbed or angry about someone close to you.

2 Say out loud what it is that upset you, making sure that you are completely honest with yourself and without judging. For example:
"You are always so (needy/ demanding/condescending …) and you never (respect my space/ pay attention when I talk/give me a chance to prove I can be independent)."

3 Then change the word "you" for the word "I" and say the sentence out loud again: *"I am always so (needy) and I never (respect your space)."*
Try to be open and really willing to feel the true meaning of what you say and note how it makes you feel.

4 Repeat the sentence from Step 3 three times. and see what emotions come up, if any. If strong feelings do arise, simply let them happen.

5 To finish the exercise, write down any insights you have to deepen your awareness of the experience.

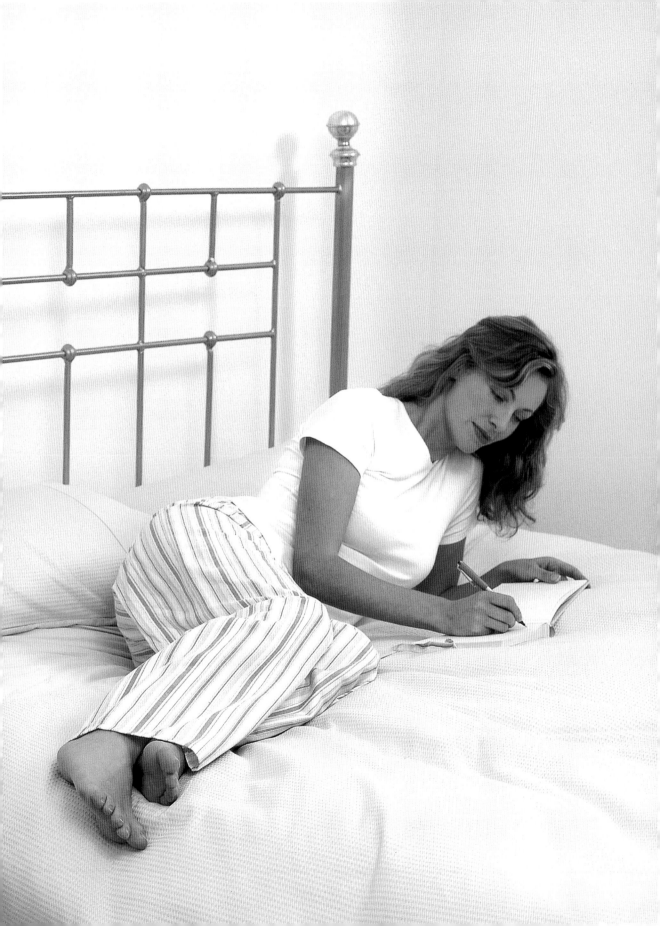

Supporting intimacy

INTIMACY SIMPLY MEANS being open and vulnerable to another person – willing to share your thoughts, feelings and energy. This is often easier said than done as many people are afraid to open up, fearing that they will be hurt and so choosing to stay safe in their closed shell. However, only people with an open heart can receive love and harmony into their lives.

Treating the heart chakra (see p. 140) with Reiki enhances feelings of inner joy and contentment, encouraging you to love yourself more and, in turn, deepening your relationships with loved ones around you. Reiki is particularly useful at times when words seem inadequate to express the depths of your love: touch can be used to remind us of that which is deeply felt – at our cores – and can remind us to love others as they are.

Reiki can also be used to treat problems you may encounter with sexual intimacy, such as impotence or a lack of sexual desire. Such problems may be due to a fear of intimacy – of "exposing" ourselves so openly – in which case giving yourself a daily Reiki treatment, such as the one below, is of great benefit. It could alternatively be a sign that there are other areas in your relationship that need attention (see exercises such as *OSHO Nadabrahma Meditation for Couples*, p. 45, and *Talking & Listening*, p. 46). However, you should always consult a medical doctor first to determine whether there are any physical reasons.

Sexual Problems:
Self-treatment

This treatment helps to balance the energy of the first chakra (linked to the reproductive organs), the second chakra (the centre of vitality and sensuality) and the "third eye" (linked to the pineal and pituitary glands and lower brain). Remain in each treatment position for about three to five minutes. (See p. 140 for chakra positions.)

"Reiki helped me to connect on an emotional level with my partner, "unsticking" a certain aspect of our relationship and renewing our sex life."

SUE, 38, REIKI TRAINEE

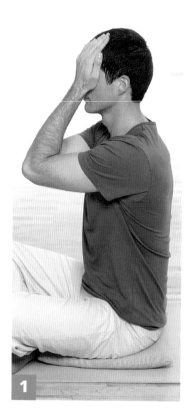

1

1 Place your hands over your eyes (see also Head Position 1, p. 18).

2 Then place your hands over the back of the head, over the medulla oblongata (see also Head Position 4, p. 19).

3 Move your hands to Front Position 1, with both hands pointing inwards on the chest (see p. 20).

4 Use Front Position 3, with the hands on the belly (see p. 20).

5 Next, use Front Position 4 (see pp. 15 and 20).

6 Use Back Position 3, with the fingers pointing towards the spine on the lower middle back (see p. 21).

7 Then finish with your fingers on the coccyx pointing downwards and inwards on the sacrum (see also Back Position 4, p. 21).

SUPPORTING INTIMACY**4 3**

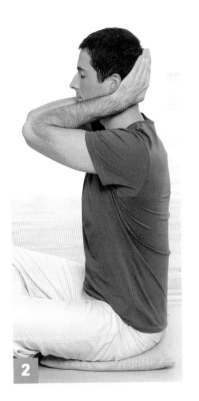

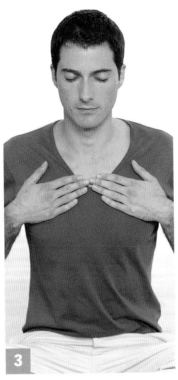

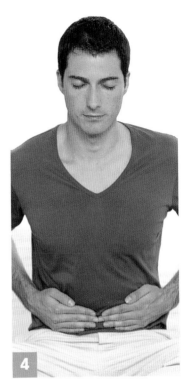

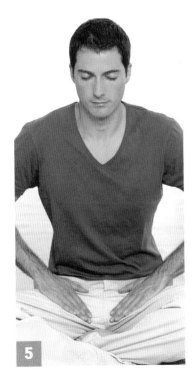

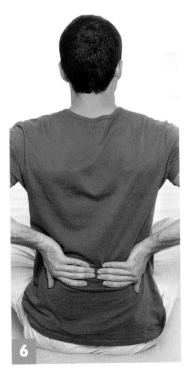

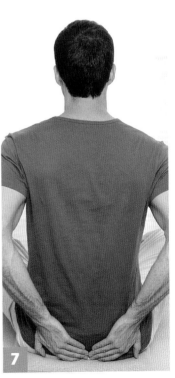

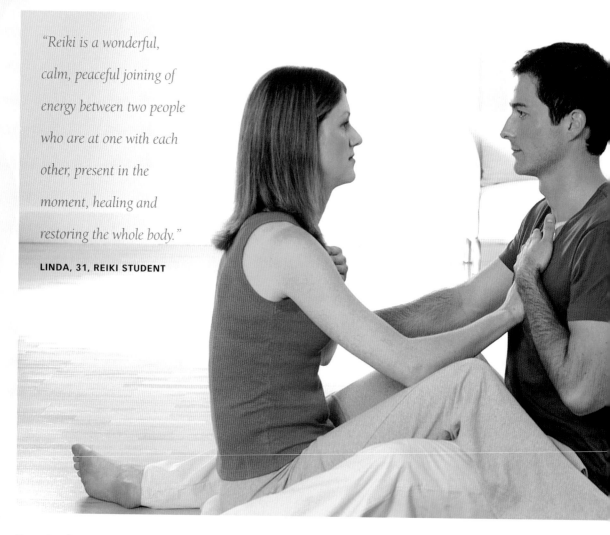

"Reiki is a wonderful, calm, peaceful joining of energy between two people who are at one with each other, present in the moment, healing and restoring the whole body."

LINDA, 31, REIKI STUDENT

Developing Closeness

If you and your partner have had an argument and are ready to make up, try this exercise. Alternatively, do the exercise when you feel you haven't had much quality time together recently or are feeling quite disconnected from one another. You can play gentle music while doing it if you like. You could even try the exercise during lovemaking in order to experience your sexuality on a deeper level, suffused with feelings of love, tenderness, trust, caring and unity.

1 Sit face to face, close enough that you can each comfortably reach your partner's chest. Use cushions to make you feel at ease.

2 Each of you should lay your right hand on your partner's heart centre and your left hand over his or her hand on your own chest. Drop your chin, keep your breathing relaxed and allow the Reiki energy to flow into the chest area while gazing gently into each other's eyes.

3 After one or two minutes both of you should close your eyes. Stay for as long as you like in this position – perhaps for fifteen to twenty minutes. You may feel a strong sense of love and unity.

OSHO Nadabrahma Meditation for Couples

This meditation is a variation of the one shown on p. 137, developed by the contemporary mystic, Osho. It is based on an old Tibetan technique and supports the balance of giving and receiving – an important part of intimate relationships. You should allow an hour to do it at any time of the day when you will not be disturbed. When the partner is of the opposite sex, the meditation is enhanced by the exchange of male and female energies that takes place, but same-sex couples can gain great benefit from it, too.

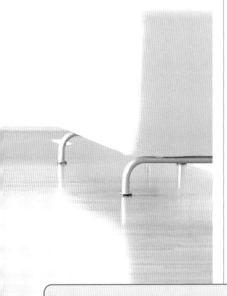

1 Sit comfortably facing your partner, holding each other's crossed hands. Close your eyes and hum together for 30 minutes. Humming together helps the energies of both partners to merge and unite. Feel your energies melting into each other as the vibration of the humming fills your body.

2 Keeping your eyes closed, let go of your partner's hands and bring your hands to your own body, palms facing upwards just in front of the navel. Then slowly move your hands in wide, flat circles, outwards from the navel to each side of your body. Keep the movement of the hands and arms very slow and conscious for 7$\frac{1}{2}$ minutes. Feel how you are giving out energy in the direction of your partner.

3 Now turn your palms down towards the floor and reverse the direction of the circles you make with your hands, bringing them back towards your body, again for 7$\frac{1}{2}$ minutes. Feel yourself receiving energy.

4 Keeping your eyes closed, lie down on your back and remain absolutely still and silent for fifteen minutes. You may prefer to lie on your side and place one leg over and one leg under your partner's legs. Gently hold your partner's legs wherever feels most comfortable for both of you.

Suggestion: If you and your partner are comfortable with it, you could choose to do this meditation naked and cover both your bodies loosely with a sheet, like a tent. You could also light candles and burn incense, if you like.

Connecting with your Child

The *Developing Closeness* exercise is also a great way to deepen your bond with your child. It can be done sitting, as above, but it is particularly nice to do it lying down, facing one another, as this is a very nurturing position.

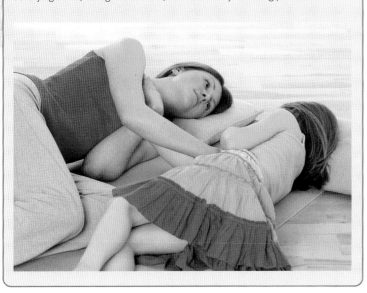

Sharing

MOST OF US LONG TO HAVE nourishing relationships. We can easily share our energy and happiness with our loved ones, but it is also important to share our tears, anger or other potentially negative feelings and thoughts that we have been holding back. When we can talk about our hurt feelings and expose ourselves even in times of sadness, pain or anger, the sharing in itself has a tremendous healing power. We also show our partner that we trust them by exposing ourselves. Just knowing that our partner is listening will make us feel understood. This creates deep intimacy between us and our partner.

Talking and Listening

This exercise is particularly helpful when you have a conflict with a friend or partner and you need to talk, clarify a situation and/or share your feelings, but you do not want to end up arguing. A "speaking tool" is used to signify the role of the speaker. This can be any item, as its purpose is simply to empower the holder with the chance to speak freely and uninterrupted, and to remind the listener that it is not yet their turn to speak. Although it involves no actual hands-on Reiki, this technique is a wonderful way to connect on a deeper level with another person. It is recommended not to let it exceed a total time of one hour.

> *If you are attuned to the* **Reiki Second Degree**, *you can use the First Reiki symbol to enhance awareness during the talk and strengthen the energy. Draw or visualise the Reiki symbol between you and your partner.*

1 First, agree on the length of time for which you each want to speak – equal amounts of time, such as five or ten minutes each, is preferable – and decide on who is going to speak first.

2 The first speaker should then take the "speaking tool" and begin to speak about whatever is on their mind, be it frustration, disappointment or

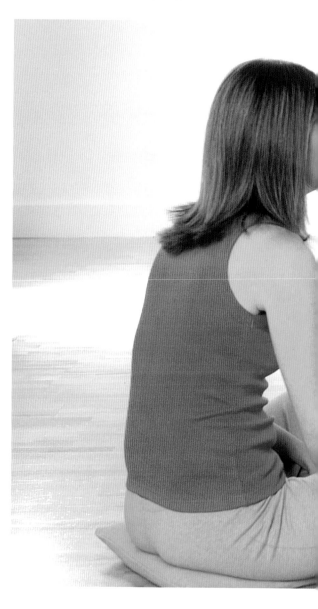

confusion about a recent interaction, *"I often find myself overwhelmed with too many little jobs to do around the house, which makes me feel stressed and undervalued."* or *"I miss spending time with you."* The other person simply listens from the heart without interrupting or responding. Their aim is really to listen from the heart and try to absorb what the other person has to

say. However tempting it might be to start mentally defending yourself, gently stop yourself from thinking about what you will say when it is your turn.

3 When the speaker is finished, they should place the speaking tool between the two of you, and the other person should pick it up to take over the role of the speaker. The new listener should

then try to listen attentively and fully from the heart. This switching of speaking/listening roles can be repeated two or three more times within one sitting if necessary.

Suggestion: This exercise usually works best if the listener keeps track of the time.

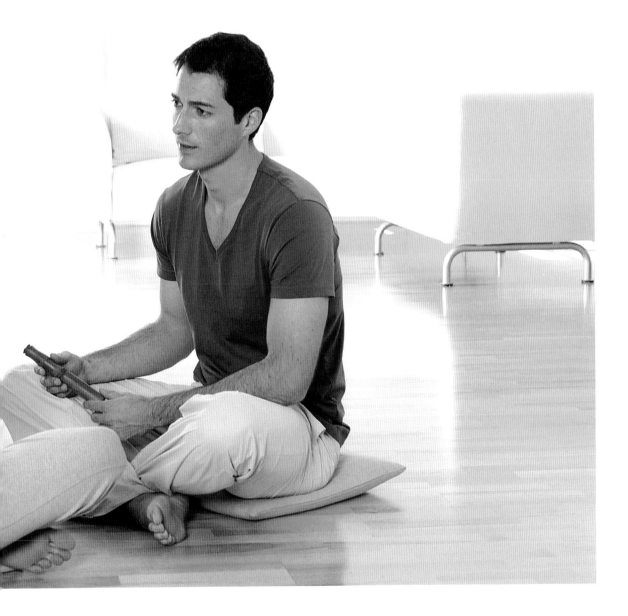

Accepting

PEOPLE IN RELATIONSHIPS often have expectations about themselves and their loved ones. Each expects the other to make them "happy". Perhaps it's to keep us company, to be there when we need them or to support us in our dealings with other people. Whatever our expectations of the other person, all "expecting" will ultimately bring disappointment, as others can only be the way they are. When we set up a condition and it is not fulfilled, we are hurt. The usual reaction is to blame others and become angry or frustrated at them for not fulfilling our needs, rather than looking within ourselves for the root causes of our unhappiness. When we can look at the events in our lives as an opportunity for learning and inner growth, we are no longer a victim. We take responsibility for the events happening in our life and we might be able to see the simplicity in accepting things and people as they are. We are ready to see that nothing actually needs to change to make us happy and content. Richness is available in each and every moment.

Having said that, anger and all other strong emotions are a natural part of life, and they are important to acknowledge as they arise. Otherwise, layers of such emotion could build up, causing repression and, potentially, great sadness, pain and depression. Reiki can help you, first, to recognise underlying emotions and, second, to balance and transform these feelings into positive ones.

Dealing with Anger and Frustration

Receiving this treatment relaxes you and allows your emotional energies to come back into balance. Treating the kidneys and adrenal glands (as shown in Step 4) also calms and strengthens your nerves, allowing you to let go more easily. If tears come up, just let them flow and keep your hands in the position where the emotion started until the feeling dissolves. Otherwise, keep your hands in each position for about five minutes. You can play relaxing music in the background if you wish.

1 The receiver should lie down comfortably with their eyes closed. Suggest to them that they take a few deep breaths, relaxing with each out-breath.

2 Lay both your hands on the top of the head, leaving a gap between the hands to avoid the sensitive crown chakra area (see p. 140). This helps to centre the receiver and to release stress.

3 Next, place your hands around the throat, without directly touching it. This is good for repressed anger and frustration and promotes balanced self-expression.

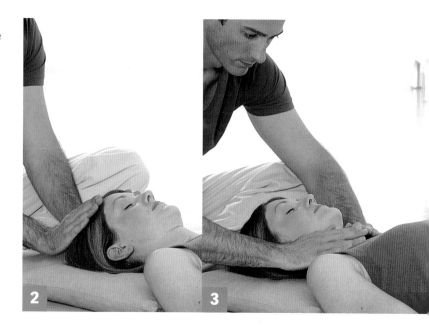

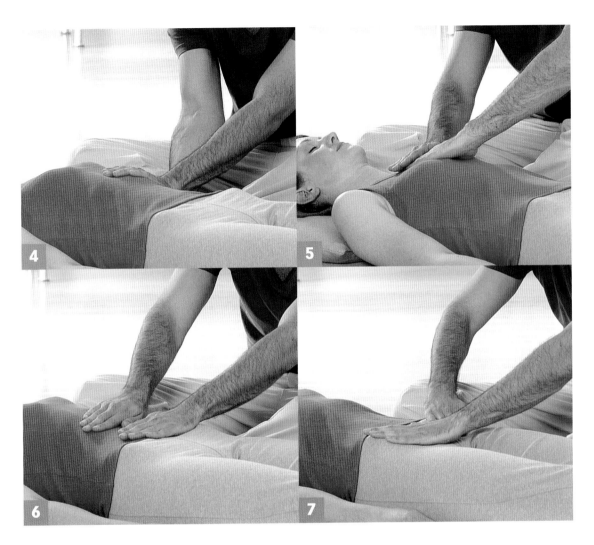

4 Place one hand on the lower left side of the ribcage and the other under the body where the kidneys and adrenals are located – on the left side of the middle back. This calms strong emotions and releases stress and pain. Now walk around the receiver and treat them in the same way from the right side of the body – one hand on the lower right side of the ribcage and the other under the middle back. This helps to reduce fear and frustration, and balances emotions such as anger and depression.

5 Place one hand on the breastbone and the other across the thymus gland, below the collarbone: the hands should form a T shape (Front Position 1, see p. 14). This promotes relaxation, allows the emotional energies to come back into balance and helps to increase the capacity for love and the enjoyment of life.

6 Place one hand above and the other below the navel. Doing this is calming and releases powerful emotions, such as fear, depression and shock.

7 Lay both hands over the lower abdomen in the shape of a V, with your hands touching over the pubic bone when treating a female (see p. 20), or wider, over the groin area, when treating a male (see p. 15). This position provides grounding and helps to relieve existential fear.

Dealing with Anger & Frustration: Self-treatment

This treatmeant is a variation of the one on pages 48–9 that you can apply to yourself.

1 Lay one hand on the forehead and the other over the medulla oblongata at the back of the head.

2 Then lay your hands around your throat, wrists touching at the centre and fingertips pointing backwards.

3 Next, lay your left hand underneath the left side of your middle back, fingertips pointing towards the spine, where the kidneys and adrenals are located. Place the right hand over the lower left side of the front ribcage. If you are doing the exercise lying down, you may want to support your right arm with a small cushion under your elbow. Then do the same on the right side of the body, this time with the right hand on the back of the body and the left hand on the front.

4 Place one hand on the middle of the chest and the other on the breastbone underneath the collarbone.

5 Lay one hand above the navel, covering your solar plexus and the other hand below the navel, touching your stomach.

6 Lay both hands over the lower abdomen in the shape of a V, with your hands touching over the pubic bone for a female (see p. 20) or wider, over the groin area, for a male (see p. 15).

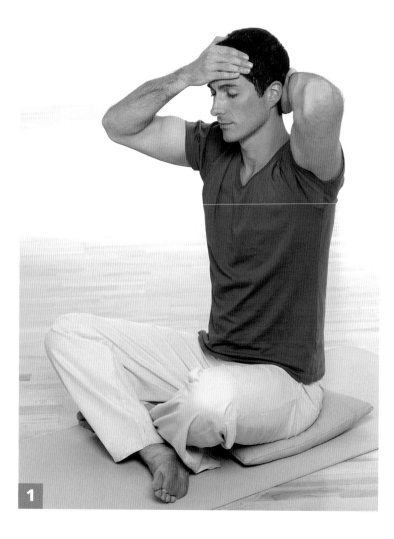

1

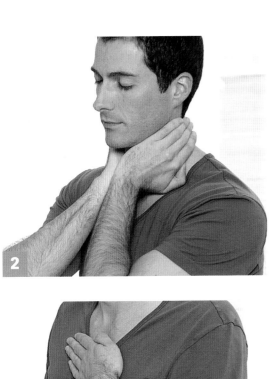

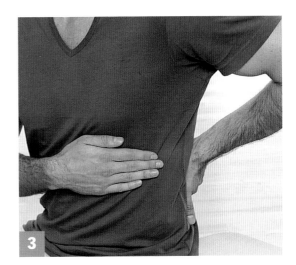

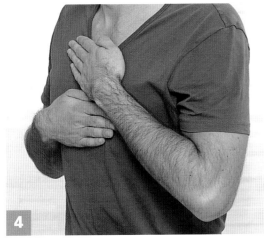

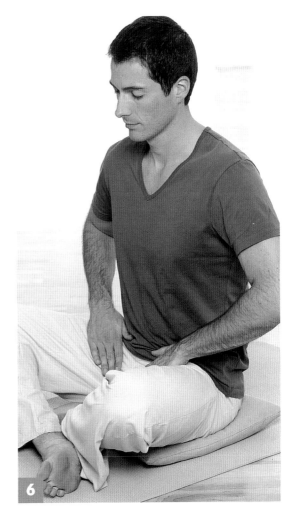

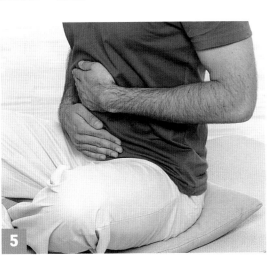

Treating children

ALL CHILDREN ARE FULL OF LIFE ENERGY when they are born, which means they are much closer to "the source" – to God – than adults, most of whom have forgotten their divine connection. Children have not had the necessary time to build up the same barriers, belief systems and self-defence mechanisms as adults.

However, children are intelligent, sensitive beings who learn from whatever surrounds them, so it is important that they are brought up in a safe environment by loving, trustworthy parents in order to have a strong, healthy foundation for the rest of life. As parents, our first responsibility is, therefore, to be respectful and understanding towards our children, trusting them,

supporting their potential and creativity, and giving them freedom to be themselves. When we accept that our children have come through us, but do not belong to us, we realise that they have their own destiny. By respecting our children we can learn a lot from them, just the way they are.

Reiki is an extremely effective means of helping children to release stress, to balance their overactive energies, to give them support with any learning difficulties and also to help them to deal with strong emotions, such as frustration, anger, sadness or mood swings. On a physical level, Reiki also helps to strengthen their immune system.

Calming Overactive Energies

Giving your children Reiki before falling asleep can be a valuable ritual for you all, so as long as your children allow you to put them to bed, you should do this exercise. It helps to ease any fears and worries that might arise from their dreams during the night, and makes them feel cosy and protected. You can also sing a child a song, tell a calming story or play soft music in the background to lull them further into a sense of peace and security.

1 Once your child is in bed, ask her to close her eyes and then smooth down the aura by slowly moving both your hands a little above the body – from the top of the head down, over the whole body, to the feet.

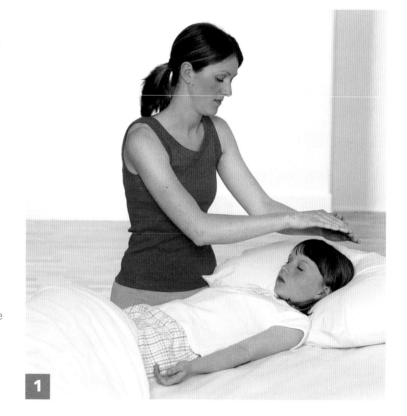

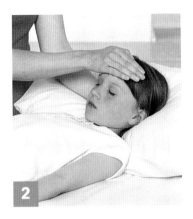

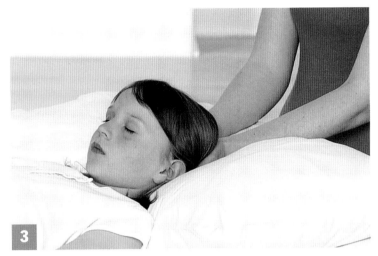

2 Place one hand on the back of the head, over the medulla oblongata, and the other hand on the middle of the forehead, covering the third eye (sixth chakra; see p. 140). This position is calming and releases stress.

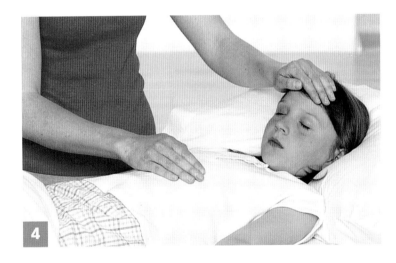

3 Cup the back of the head, with your palms over the medulla oblongata – between the head and the neck. This will help your child to fall asleep more easily and create a feeling of security.

4 Place one hand over the child's forehead and the other on the solar plexus (third chakra; see p. 140) in order to harmonise and balance emotional energies.

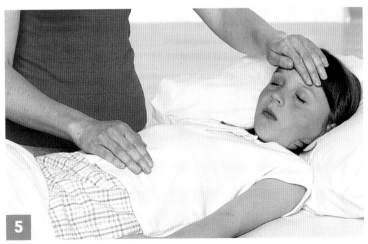

5 Keep one hand on the forehead and move the other hand down onto the stomach. This position generates a feeling of deep relaxation.

Suggestion: You can also use Step 5 as a single treatment to aid sleep, in which case you should keep your hands in that position for about ten minutes, or until your child falls asleep.

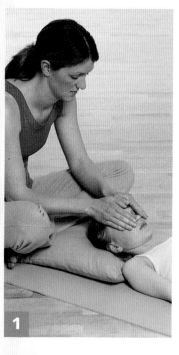

1

Helping with Concentration & Learning Difficulties

This treatment helps your child to concentrate better – especially useful before an exam – and activates the long- and short-term memory. It also helps ease stress and excessive mental activity. You may choose to give the treatment in silence or play soothing music in the background. Allow between ten and fifteen minutes, or as long as it feels right.

1 Once the child is lying or sitting down, place your hands over the eyes, forehead and cheeks to help energy to move back inwards. A lot of energy usually moves out through the eyes when they are open, so relaxing the eyes relaxes the whole body.

2 Now lay your hands on each side of your child's head, fingertips touching the temples and palms following the shape of the head. This position balances the right (intuitive) and left (logical) side of the brain, and helps with learning and concentration difficulties.

3 Finally, lay your hands on the back of the head, holding it like a ball, in order to release tension and ease powerful emotions, such as fear.

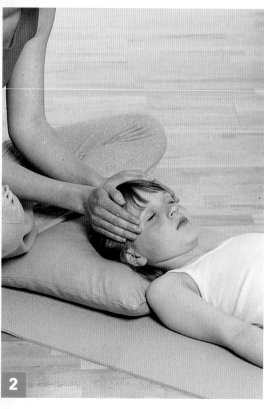

2

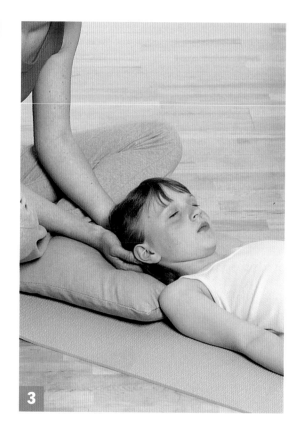

3

Treating Mood Swings & the Blues

Treating your child's head with Reiki helps to increase the production of endorphins – the body's "happiness hormones" – and giving Reiki to the solar plexus and middle back reinforces confidence and self-esteem. Allow between fifteen and twenty minutes, or as long as is needed, for this treatment.

1 Place your hands on either side of the head, fingertips touching the temples and the palms following the shape of the head. This position calms the mind and encourages your child to reconnect with a feeling of joy in life.

2 Cup the back of the head with your palms, fingertips over the medulla oblongata between the head and the neck. This position strengthens intuition and brings clarity.

3 Place one hand on each side of the lower front ribcage. This treats the solar plexus, increasing energy, promoting relaxation, and reducing any fears and frustration.

4 Ask your child to turn over onto their front and place your hands on the back of the waist, at kidney height, to strengthen the kidneys, adrenal glands and nerves. This will help the receiver let go of stress, fear and pain.

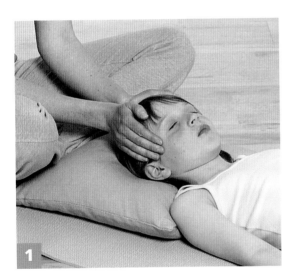

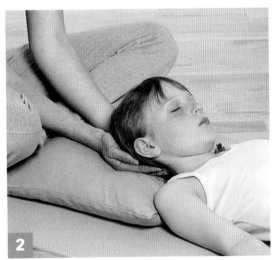

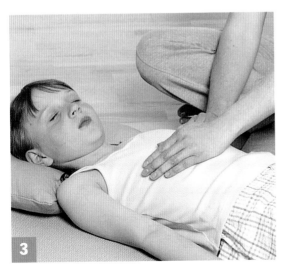

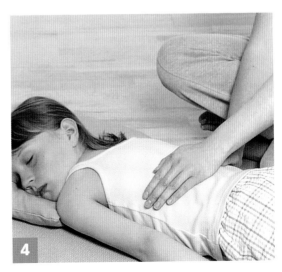

Treating babies

TREATING BABIES WITH REIKI is very effective as they are so full of energy, contented and connected to "the source". In fact, just touching and carrying your baby as much as possible is a form of Reiki in that it "feeds" him or her with light and energy, as well as opening your own heart energy.

However, you can also give your baby short daily Reiki treatments, such as the ones suggested below. Giving your child Reiki is likely to deepen the bond between you, thus enhancing your own emotional well-being, too.

We usually do not need to give babies full treatments – between ten and twenty minutes tend to be enough. They will often roll to the side or crawl away when they have taken enough energy. Trust your intuition about where to place your hands and for how long.

If you sense that your baby does not respond well to direct touch, simply keep your hands a little above the body – the energy will be absorbed just as well. Reiki can be particularly useful to calm babies when they seem nervous or restless, have wind, are experiencing pain when teething or are having problems getting to sleep. You can also treat babies with Reiki while they are asleep, for example, if they appear to be slightly restless.

Sleep Help

Place one hand on the forehead and the other hand over the belly to help your baby fall asleep more quickly.

Easy Treatments

• If your baby is **lying on his side**, place one hand on the back of the head and the other hand on the back itself. This way you cover almost the whole torso and all the energy centres, and balance and harmonise the energies.

• If your baby is **lying on his back**, place one hand underneath the baby's back and the other on the tummy.

• If your baby is **lying on his tummy**, place one hand underneath the tummy and the other over the back. This position harmonises the energy.

Both options 2 and 3 mean that your child lies between both of your hands and receives healing energy throughout the whole body. You are also treating all the organs, which helps digestive problems, such as wind or diarrhoea.

Case study

Baby Tobias was recuperating from meningitis, but it was taking a long time for him to lose his high temperature and the spots on his body. The day after receiving a Reiki treatment his temperature dropped and within three days he had regained his usual energy. His parents also reported that he seemed to experience a "developmental spurt", making up for the time lost through illness.

"Your children are not your children.

They are the sons and daughters of Life's longing for itself.

They come through you but not from you,

And though they are with you, yet they belong not to you.

You may give them your love but not your thoughts,

For they have their own thoughts.

You may house their bodies but not their souls,

For their souls dwell in the house of tomorrow, which you cannot

visit, not even in your dreams."

KAHLIL GIBRAN
***THE PROPHET*, 1923**

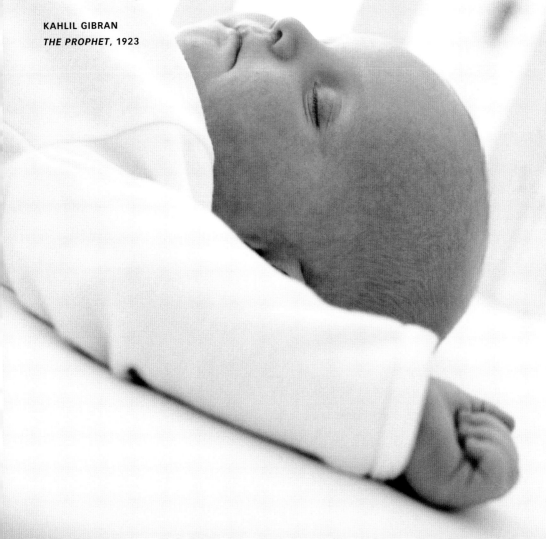

Treating older people

LIVING CONDITIONS have changed much over the past few decades and are likely to continue to do so. The traditional family structure has gradually weakened, and older people can feel disoriented with the fast pace of the modern world around them. The deepest hurt and disturbance often happens when they feel undervalued and useless, especially by a society that increasingly idealises youth and is obsessed with the "new". Our Western culture tries hard to ignore the fact that we will all get old and one day die. As long as we do not accept death as a reality and a part of life we will have a deep fear of old age and dying.

Older people can gain immense benefit from regular physical contact, including massage and Reiki treatments.

The warmth of the hands on their bodies helps to lessen any pain or discomfort, especially if they are living alone or in a hospice where they might not have much physical contact with others. Nowadays there are more and more people in the caring professions who know about and are trained in Reiki for this reason.

Giving Reiki to elderly members of your family nourishes and energises them and also imparts healing and strength to your relationships, as it creates the space for a silent connection from heart to heart. It is a special gift to be able to give Reiki to your own parents or grandparents. And the fact that Reiki energy is not hindered by clothing is also an advantage.

Short Treatments

It can often be best to give elderly people Reiki in a sitting position for maximum comfort. The first two treatments should be short – between 20 and 30 minutes (see the example treatment on the right) – so that the person can become accustomed to the healing energy. A long treatment may put a strain on an older person, so trust your own insight and intuition about the length of the treatment and always check with the receiving person. After giving two to three shorter treatments, you might want to give a full body treatment (see pp. 12–17), which usually lasts about one hour.

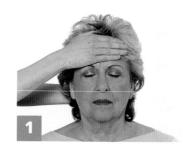

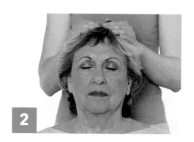

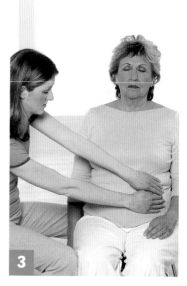

1 Place one hand over the receiver's forehead and the other on the back of the head – over the medulla oblongata.

2 Place both hands gently on top of the receiver's head – over the crown chakra

– leaving a gap between your hands to avoid touching.

3 Then place your hands on the receiver's belly, one side at a time, to help the digestion.

Pain in the Joints

Arthritis is a particularly common disorder in the later years. It is an inflammation of the joints and its typical characteristics are swelling, redness, pain and extreme stiffness. Osteoarthritis is the common "wear-and-tear" form that causes so many aches and pains; and rheumatoid arthritis, which occurs mostly in women, is an auto-immune disorder in which the immune system attacks the body's joints as it would an invading bacteria or virus. However, there are different types of arthritis, many of which are caused by bacteria and viruses, such as infective arthritis.

It is important to consult a medical doctor to see how they can help you deal with your symptoms. However, it is also worth bearing in mind that the disorder can be partially due to emotional imbalances, such as overly rigid thinking, being excessively critical of oneself or feeling unloved. Reiki can help with both these physical and emotional elements.

1 Ask the receiver to sit or lie down, and find out where they feel the most pain. Then hold your hands directly on these areas. It is best if you sandwich the joint concerned, with one hand above and the other hand below it.

2 If the receiver feels comfortable, you can then treat the entire body (see *Full Reiki treatment*, pp. 12–17).

3 Next, place one hand on the upper leg, where it joins the buttocks, and the other hand on the heel. It is easiest to do this if the receiver lies on their stomach – but only if they feel comfortable lying in this position.

4 Finally, lay your hands on the soles of the feet, fingertips pointing down. This treats the foot reflex zones for all the body's regions and energises the feet.

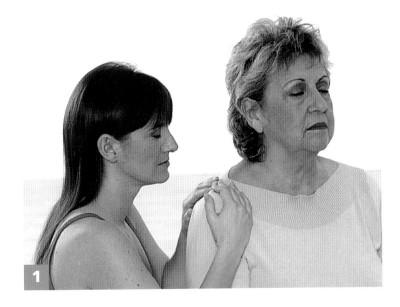

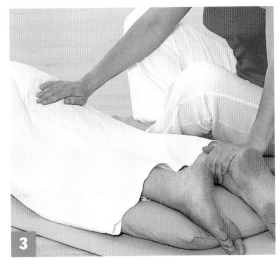

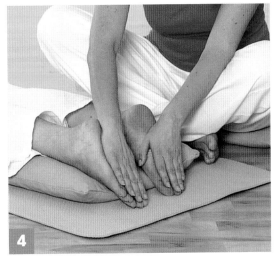

Treating pets & plants

MOST ANIMALS SEEM TO LOVE receiving Reiki. When your pet is unwell, you can help it to feel better and boost its immune system simply by laying on hands and giving Reiki. They sense immediately that something special is being given to them, as well as just enjoying the attention.

The placement of organs in all mammals, including humans, is very similar, so specific treatment positions are also similar. When an animal knows you, it will often show you by its body position where to place your hands, such as a dog rolling onto its back to urge you to place your hands on its belly. It will also often let you know when it's had enough by changing position or standing up to leave, but from ten to thirty minutes is usually about right.

> **CASE STUDY**
> *After a vaccination by the vet, the dog of a Reiki trainee developed a serious inflammation in the area that had been injected. It became as big as a tennis ball and the vet suggested that it needed to be surgically removed. Reluctant to agree to this without first trying an alternative, the owner started giving Reiki to the affected area for a half hour each evening for three weeks. The inflamed area returned to normal again and no operation was needed.*

Treating Pets

• Treat behind the ears or place one hand on top of the head and the other under the throat to generally comfort your pet.

• Treat the chest, stomach, back and/or hips for any ailments – from stomach upsets to arthritis.

• Treat painful spots directly – over the plaster in the case of broken bones.

• For fish: place your hands around the tank or over the pond.

• For birds: place your hands around either the bird or the cage.

• Holding your pet while in the waiting room at the vet's, channelling Reiki energy to them through your hands, will often help to calm them and ease their fears. If possible, also place your hands on them during the examination.

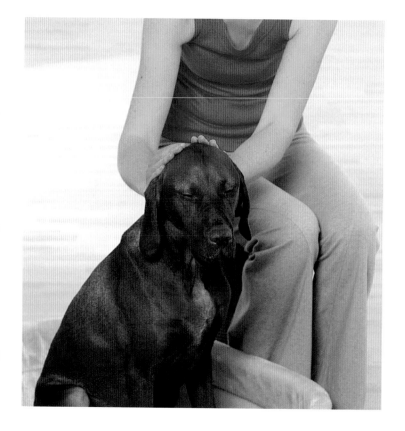

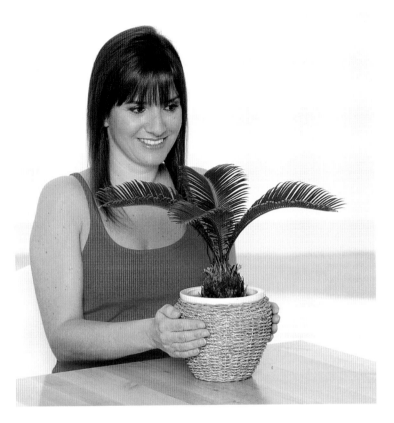

Treating Plants

We all like our plants and flowers to look healthy and vibrant, as they can make such a difference to the environment in which we live – bringing nature and extra life into our homes. Plants and flowers – whether indoor or outdoor – can be given Reiki treatments in just the same way as people – whether to help them stay healthy, grow faster or recover from a specific problem. Simply hold them in your hands or place your hands above or around them for a few moments, mindfully transferring Universal Life Energy to them.

• Treat seeds with Reiki before planting them. Several days after planting, give Reiki again by placing your hands over the soil.

• Place your hands around the roots of seedlings or plants before planting.

• Treat the roots of potted plants by putting your hands around the pot. Treat the leaves by placing your hands around the leaves.

• When you repot a plant, treat the roots before putting it in its new container.

• Treat cut flowers by placing your hands around the stems and later around the vase.

• Encourage herbs and vegetables to grow stronger and more quickly by placing your hands around them.

• Treat your entire garden with the Distant Healing technique (see p. 139) – particularly useful when you are on holiday or have just sown seeds and are waiting for a good harvest.

If it is not possible to treat animals directly, **Second Degree practitioners** *can use the Distant Healing technique (see p.139) to help bring them healing and comfort. This can be particularly useful if you want to treat animals who live at the zoo or in shelters.*

CASE STUDY

Horses are very sensitive animals and they seem to love Reiki energy. Richard, a Reiki trainee and horse owner, told me that whenever there is a problem with his horse, such as a sore joint or a muscle strain, he holds his hands directly around the affected area for ten to twenty minutes. He also lays his hands on the horse's forehead and behind the ears. When he does this, he notices the horse become visibly calmer – as if enjoying the healing energy.

Chapter 3

Work Life

"When you work with love you bind yourself to yourself, and to one another. And what is it to work with love? It is to weave the cloth with threads drawn from your heart, even as if your beloved were to wear that cloth. It is to charge all things you fashion with a breath of your own spirit."

KAHLIL GIBRAN, *THE PROPHET*, 1923

WE ARE LIVING IN FAST-CHANGING TIMES, and technological developments in the last few decades have changed most of our working conditions, as well as the way we communicate with each other. However, the technology and computers that help us at work also challenge us with new tasks, bombard us with seemingly endless amounts of information and mean that we are almost always expected to be "on call", whether via mobile phones or e-mails. We are also under pressure to be flexible with our time and to be able to balance many activities at the same time, and this multi-tasking can be overwhelming.

The problem is that we usually cannot release the stress that we experience at work straight away. If we have an argument with the boss, for example, it's not an option to get visibly angry or walk away. Although we might feel like it, our human conditioning does not allow such behaviour and we would also run the risk of being fired. So we usually keep quiet, swallowing our anger. In this way we are holding stress and anger in the body, which can manifest itself as physical tensions, pain and even illness.

Other life forms do not hold onto such stress and tension. For example, if you watch two ducks having a fight, they release the tension immediately afterwards by flapping their wings two or three times and they then go on swimming as though nothing has happened. But we humans do hold on to stress. We worry about all manner of things, from maybe not being capable or intelligent enough to fulfil a new task that has been given to us, to whether or not our new boss will like us.

Most people develop unconscious coping mechanisms for dealing with stressful situations. Some people eat or drink too much, smoke excessively or feel lethargic and stop exercising. Others experience symptoms like nervousness, anxiety attacks, fatigue, low spirits, mood swings, sudden sweating, forgetfulness, aggression, depression, frustration or dissatisfaction. Some of these symptoms might even develop into disorders such as dermatitis, asthma, migraine or a gastric ulcer. Even high blood pressure, heart trouble, diabetes and sterility can have their origins in stress.

Reiki is a means of relieving all the stress and pain, as well as getting right to the root cause of the stress symptoms and supporting us in finding ways to prevent stress becoming a problem in the first place. For example, it encourages us to trust ourselves more and reconnects us with our creativity and feelings of joy and enthusiasm

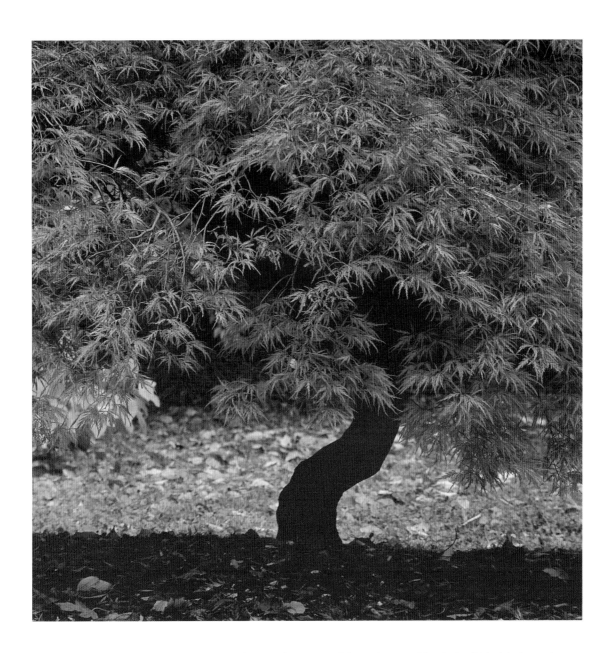

for life, which in turn give us a more relaxed and productive attitude to work. Reiki can also be a useful tool to help us to improve relations with our work colleagues – by helping our communication skills to move onto a deeper level. It also enables us to remain in the present moment with our work, rather than thinking and worrying ahead too much, thus increasing job satisfaction.

All these themes will be dealt with in this chapter's three sections: *Preventing stress* (see pp. 64–9), *Communication* (see pp. 70–3) and *Job satisfaction* (see pp. 74–9). Some of the exercises are ideal to do in the workplace – mainly the subtle ones that can be done seated or standing – while others are better done either at home in preparation for work or for relaxation after work.

Preventing stress

STRESSFUL SITUATIONS are all too common in the workplace, whether caused by tight deadlines; seemingly unreasonable colleagues; the demands we place on ourselves, and others, at the start of new projects; or the responsibility we feel if things don't turn out the way we expect. In any stress situation the adrenal glands secrete hormones into the blood, which transports them all around the body with profoundly harmful effects.

More and more people are developing stress-related symptoms these days, ranging from headaches, migraines and shoulder and neck pain to upset stomachs, insomnia and anxiety attacks.

You can use Reiki in any stressful, or even potentially stressful, type of situation because everyone has healing energy flowing through their hands – it's just a matter of tapping into it and learning how to use it. On a physical level, it strengthens the immune system and balances energies, rejuvenating you and quickly recharging your batteries. Emotionally, Reiki brings you back in touch with a feeling of peace and joy in life. It counteracts worries, fears and feelings of restlessness or low spirits. And on a mental level, Reiki connects you with your intuition, trust and creativity, bringing increased clarity to your decision-making.

Headaches & Migraines

This treatment helps to release the tension that often causes headaches and migraines. It will calm excessive mental activity, help to clarify your thought processes and stimulate the production of endorphins – the body's "happiness hormones". It is best to keep your hands in each treatment position for about three to five minutes, so allow fifteen minutes for the full treatment. The receiver can either sit or lie down – whichever is more convenient and comfortable.

1 Place one hand over the forehead and the other on the back of the head over the medulla oblongata, where the head and neck join. This helps stress reduction and facilitates meditation.

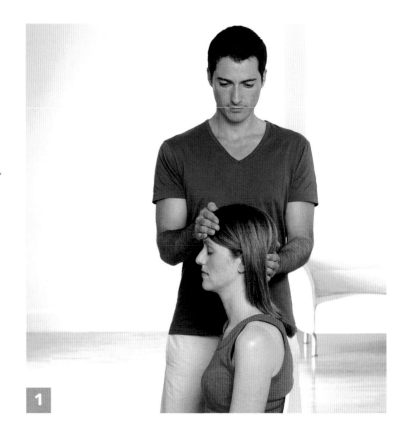

1

2 Lay your hands on either side of the head, with the base of the palms touching the temples and the fingers pointing upwards. This position treats the eye muscles and nerves, and balances the left and right sides of the brain.

3 Place the base of your palms on the back of the head, with fingers pointing upwards. This position relieves fears and calms the mind and emotions.

Suggestion: When nobody else is available to give you this treatment, you can use the same hand positions on yourself.

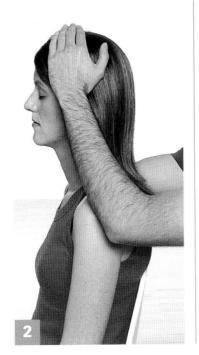

Full-body Self-treatment

If you give yourself a full-body Reiki treatment daily (see pp. 18–21), its rejuvenating effect will be noticeable: you are likely to look and feel more vibrant. It will also make you generally less susceptible to stress in the workplace, and leave you with a deep sense of well-being. The recommended self-treatment sequence should take between fifty minutes and one hour.

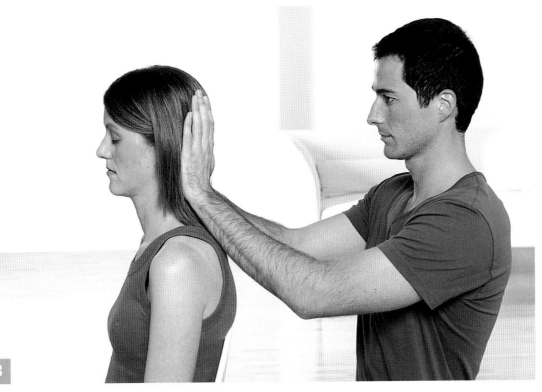

Middle & Lower Back Pain

The most common causes of middle and lower back pain are low kidney function, poor dietary habits, lack of exercise, poor posture, a lack of adequate support in life, stress and tension. Stress can disrupt the energy in the whole bodily system, but especially the muscles of the back, which go into spasm when the kidneys and related lower-back muscles weaken.

This treatment considerably eases any pain or tension in the back and is also useful to treat a hangover. It is best to keep your hands in each position for about three to five minutes. You should therefore allow about twenty to thirty minutes in total. The receiver should lie on their stomach, using cushions or towels for comfort if necessary.

1 Place both hands on the lower ribs, slightly above the waist (Back Position 3, p. 21), so that your hands are covering the adrenal glands and the upper portion of the kidneys. Then move your hands down one hand-width to cover the kidneys. Both these positions help to balance the functions of the adrenal glands, kidneys and nervous system.

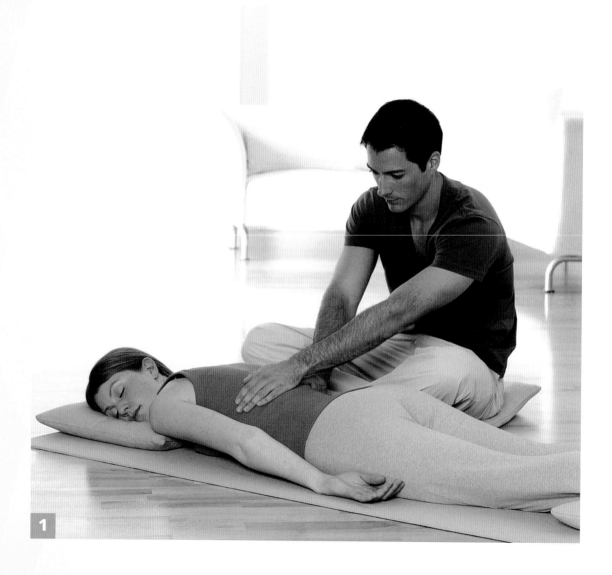

1

2 Place your hands on the lower part of the back at hip level and allow the Reiki energy to flow into this area.

3 Rest the hands on each side of the lower spine, over the sacrum area – one hand with fingertips pointing down to the tailbone and the other hand pointing upwards. Both this position and the one in Step 2 relieve sciatica and lower back pain, strengthen the lymph and nerves, and support creativity and sexuality.

4 Finish the treatment by placing one hand on the coccyx and the other hand at the top of the spine – on the neck. This balances the energy travelling along the whole spine.

Suggestion: When nobody else is available to give you this treatment, you can use the same hand positions as in Back Positions 3 and 4 (see p. 21).

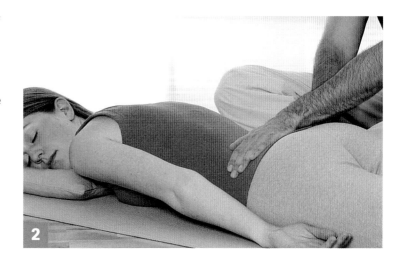

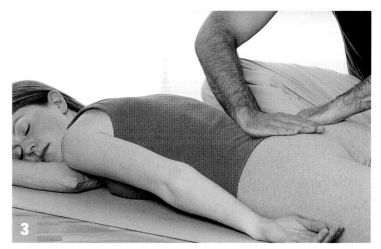

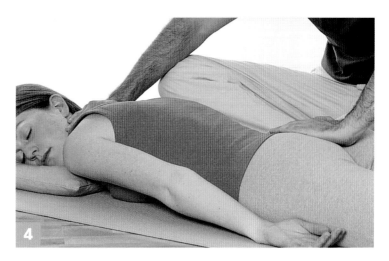

Neck & Shoulder Pain: Reiki & Massage

Tension in the neck and shoulder muscles is often caused by stress, poor posture (especially if you have to sit at a desk or computer all day), lack of exercise or imbalances in the liver and gallbladder. A feeling of being overloaded with responsibility can also cause pain in these areas.

This combination of massage and Reiki will loosen any tension in the neck, head and shoulders, and harmonise energies in the body. Total treatment time is approximately fifteen to twenty minutes. The receiver can stand or sit in any position that feels comfortable as long as the giver can easily reach their neck and shoulders.

1 Place one hand over the forehead and the other over the medulla oblongata, where the head and neck join. Stay in this position for about three minutes to help relieve feelings of exhaustion and stress.

2 Now start massaging the sides of the throat and the nape of the neck for a few minutes. Keep your touch gentle, making circular motions with your fingertips. Continue this over the medulla oblongata, on the back of the head, encouraging the receiver to sigh while exhaling to release any tension held in the body. Then massage the upper shoulders, checking with the receiver how much pressure he likes.

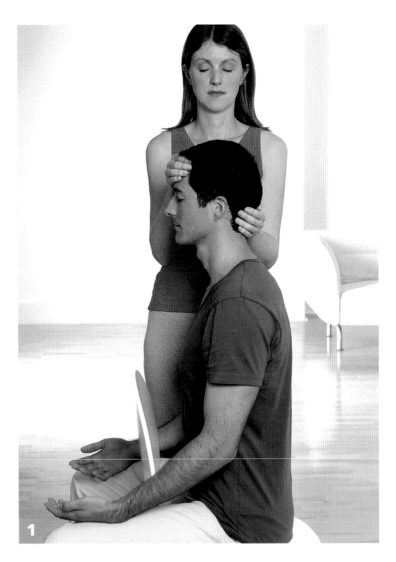

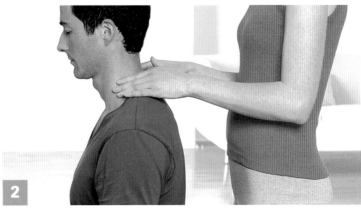

3 Place the base of your palms on the left and right sides of the upper spine, with your hands following the natural curve of the shoulders. Allow the Reiki energy to flow here for a few minutes.

4 Now massage around the shoulder blades, with circular motions of your middle and index fingers. Most of us hold a lot of tension in the area behind the shoulder blades.

5 To finish, lay one hand on the upper back between the shoulder blades and the other on the centre of the chest for a few minutes. This Reiki position strengthens the immune system.

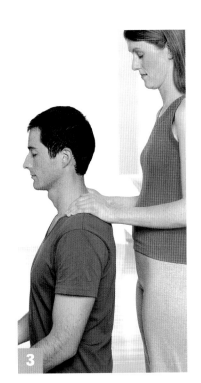

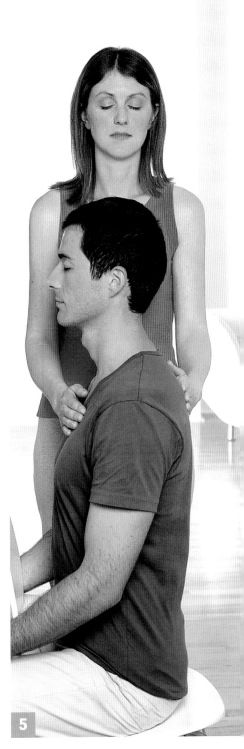

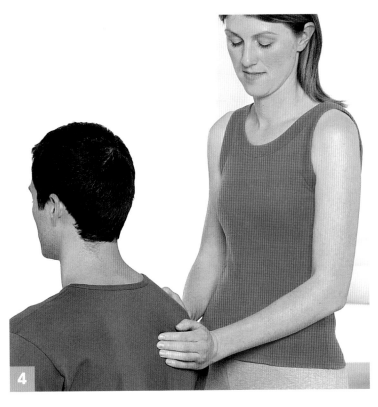

Communication

MOST COMMUNICATION of which we are aware happens through talking and listening to one another – actions of the intellect. Yet researchers studying the dynamics of communication have discovered that seventy per cent of our communication is actually non-verbal. In this sense, body language becomes very important: whether we are aware of it or not, all our movements, gestures and facial expressions are saying something about us. The spoken words are only thirty per cent of the communication.

It is important to know how to communicate effectively in the workplace – how to say things clearly so that you are not misunderstood. At the same time it is necessary to be able to listen and absorb what other people have to say. Our minds are often so loaded with our own thoughts and ideas that it can become difficult to stay present and just listen. Reiki can help you to focus your mind, stay relaxed and gain more clarity.

Giving or receiving Reiki from a colleague allows you to connect on many different levels, rather than just intellectually. The loving, healing touch – communication without words – allows you to share something special and can open up another dimension in your working relationship. This is a valuable experience, which can help you to become closer as human beings, understand each other more and therefore develop a better, more productive, working relationship.

Clearing your Head: Self-treatment

The self-treatment positions for the head (see pp. 18–19) are good for clearing your mind when you are feeling overwhelmed with thoughts, ideas and problems and are unable to prioritise effectively. However, the positions on the right can be particularly helpful to ensure that your mental faculties are functioning at their best.

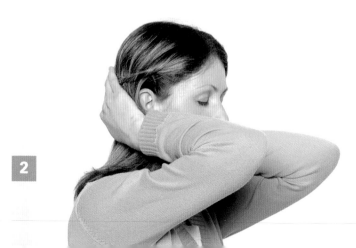

1 When you face a substantial mental challenge at work, such as giving a business presentation, leading a group discussion or developing a new project from seed, first place your hands in Head Position 2 (see p. 18).

2 Then place your hands in Head Position 4. These positions activate the short- and long-term memory (see p. 19).

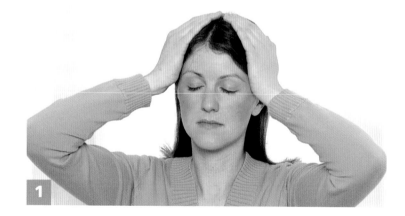

"Reiki is being able to connect with my higher self – developing my healing skills and understanding."

WILLIAM, 25, REIKI STUDENT

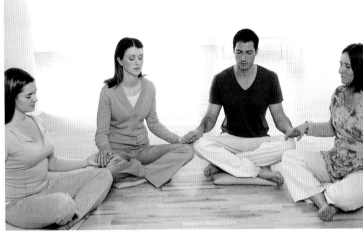

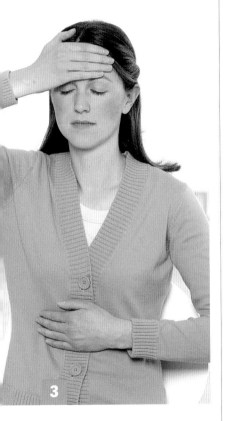

3 To clear your mind further by calming any nerves, place one hand on the solar plexus (third chakra) and the other hand on the forehead (sixth chakra). This balances any surplus energy from the head into the solar plexus area and dissipates feelings of fear.

Group Energy Circle

The fact that Reiki is a natural and effective way of transferring Universal Life Energy means we can use it to create better connections with our colleagues. For example, we could ask them to do an "energy circle" exercise, either at the beginning or the end of a group meeting or discussion, for example, to help everyone to become more present and connected. This should make everyone involved more able to share their ideas from a calm, clear position. The group energy circle usually creates close bonds among the people involved: each individual feels a part of the circle, connected with the larger whole.

1 Sit in a circle – on the floor or on chairs. Take a few deep breaths and relax your shoulders, allowing them to sink deeper with each out-breath.

2 Then hold hands with the people on either side of you so that your right palm is facing down – "giving" to the person on your right side – and your left palm is facing up – "receiving" from the person on your left. Make sure that your arms are in a comfortable position while doing this.

3 Allow the energy you receive through your left palm to pass up through your left arm, the chest area and your heart chakra (fourth energy centre) before flowing from there down your right arm and out through your right palm into the hand of the person sitting to your right. In this way, you are creating a circle of energy together.

4 Notice any sensations in your hands while giving and receiving this loving, healing energy, and become aware how you feel connected in the circle.

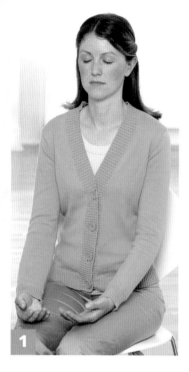
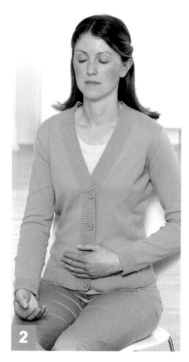
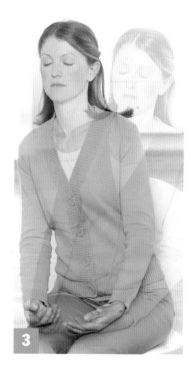
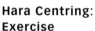

Hara Centring: Exercise

Hara is the Japanese word for the sacral chakra, which is the best known energy centre in the Eastern tradition. The Hara point, which is 5 cm (2 in) below the navel, is where we receive life energy from the cosmos, and, as such, is an important energy centre. Use this Hara-centring exercise any time you feel slightly off-centre – for example if you feel nervous about taking on a new task at work or are worried about an important meeting with your boss or colleagues. Alternatively, you can do it during your lunch break or to begin or end your working day, as it leaves you with a wonderful sense of calm and self-trust when dealing with others. And it only takes between twenty and thirty minutes.

1 Find a comfortable position to sit, with your spine straight. If you sit on a chair, make sure you keep both feet firmly on the floor and do not lean against the back. Then close your eyes and rest your hands, palms upwards, on your upper legs.

2 Visualise a line from the Hara point – 5 cm (2 in) below the navel – to the third eye chakra, between the eyebrows. Place one hand on the Hara to help to keep your attention there.

3 Start moving your upper body in an anticlockwise circle for ten to fifteen minutes. While moving, keep the torso in a straight line from the Hara point to the third eye chakra.

4 Let the circular movement become gradually smaller, until it stops completely. Then rest for about five minutes in an upright position, focusing on the energy in your Hara.

5 To finish, lie down on your back for five to ten minutes, with your arms and legs slightly open, your palms facing upwards, your mouth open slightly and your jaw relaxed.

Suggestion: You can use soothing music during the meditation to help you to relax if you like (see p. 144).

Refresh & Energise:
Self-treatment

In all our day-to-day activities we give out energy, especially when we face lots of demands at work or have a full schedule. This short Reiki treatment recharges your personal energy quickly, rejuvenating the body, mind and emotions. It is very effective after lunch or in the late afternoon, when your energy may be depleted. Total treatment time is approximately ten to fifteen minutes.

1 Find a comfortable place to sit or lie down, close your eyes and relax.

2 Place your hands over your eyes, palms on your cheekbones. Relaxing the eyes relaxes the whole body.

3 Place one hand on your solar plexus and the other beneath it, touching your stomach to restore energy and vitality.

Suggestion: You can use the same hand positions to treat another person if they are feeling low in energy and in need of a boost.

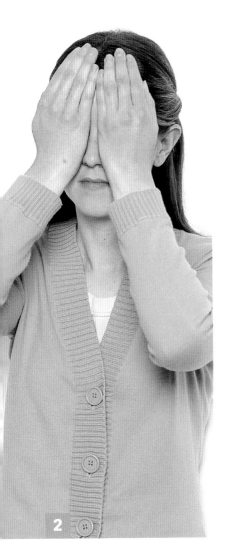

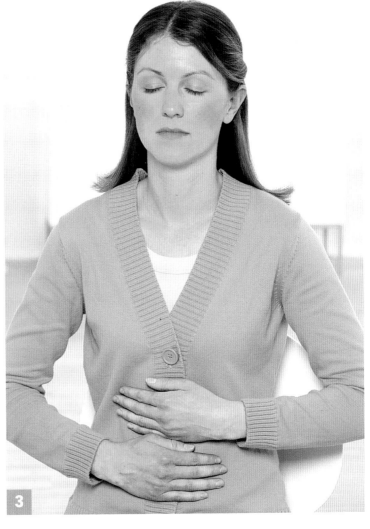

Job satisfaction

MANY PEOPLE – even when they are in jobs that they generally like – suffer from a lack of job satisfaction, which can lead to feelings of frustration and low self-esteem. There will be times, of course, when a change of role or job is needed, or when a situation with a certain person or task needs to be dealt with directly in order for change to take place. It is important, however, to recognise that the problem may often not lie so much in what you are doing, but rather in the way you are approaching your work.

Reiki will help you to become more present in your daily tasks and encourage you to relax and let go of many of the tensions you often needlessly associate with them. This may dramatically change how you view your role and therefore bring increased job satisfaction.

Reiki Self-treatment
Giving yourself a full Reiki self-treatment a few times a week greatly enhances your ability to stay relaxed in the face of chaos. See pages 18–21 for more positional guidance.

1 The five Head Positions (see p. 18–19) calm your thoughts and bring you in contact with positive qualities, such as trust, security and intuition.

2 Front Position 1 transforms negativity and increases the capacity for the enjoyment of life.

3 Front Position 2 reduces any fearful feelings and frustration.

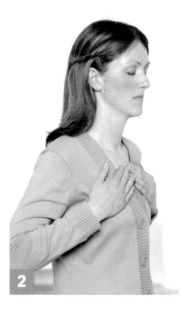

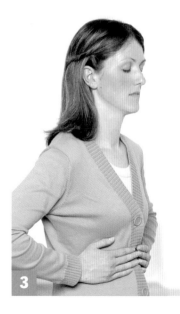

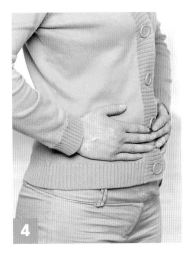

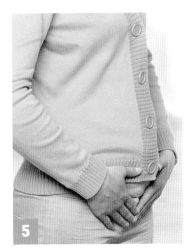

4 Front Position 3 helps to increase self-confidence.

5 Front Position 4 provides grounding and helps to eliminate fear.

6 Back Position 1 releases blocked emotions and helps any problems you have dealing with responsibility.

7 Back Position 2 helps to alleviate worries and depression. If you have difficulty reaching between your shoulder blades, place your hands on your chest, as shown in Front Position 1 (step 2).

8 Back Position 3 reinforces self-esteem and confidence.

9 Back Position 4 promotes creativity, confidence and grounding.

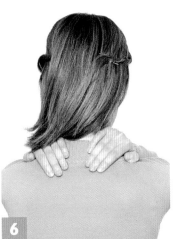

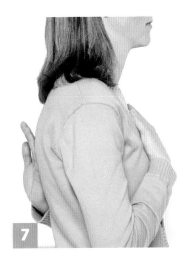

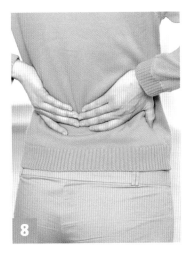

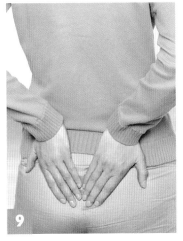

"Since practising daily Reiki there has been a tremendous amount of emotional and mental clearing in my life. I am now calmer and I feel more accepting – both in work and at home."

SARAH, 33, REIKI PRACTITIONER

Self-confidence, Power and Calm: Self-treatment

The positions shown here can be used when it is especially important for you to feel secure and confident about yourself, such as when you start a new project or take on new responsibility at work. You can also do them simply to put you in a positive mood at the start of your working day. It doesn't matter whether you sit or lie down; just stay in each treatment position for about three to five minutes.

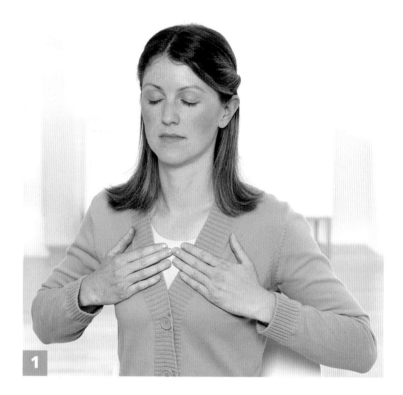

1 Place your hands next to each other on your chest (see Front Position 1, p. 20). This position stimulates the heart centre, which can transform negative emotions, helping us to accept more easily, instead of either giving in to defeat or fighting. It also strengthens the immune system and increases the capacity for the enjoyment of life.

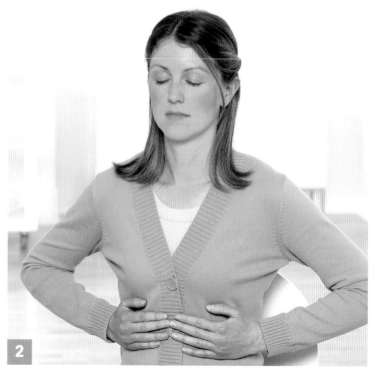

2 Now place your hands over the lower ribcage. This position gives energy, promotes relaxation and reduces fears and frustration, allowing you to trust situations more and adapt more easily to change (see Front Position 2, p. 20).

3 Place your hands on either side of the navel, fingers touching (see Front Position 3, p. 20). This position balances powerful emotions, such as fear, depression and frustration, as well as helping to increase self-confidence.

4 Place your hands on your back at waist height, fingers pointing towards the spine (see Back Position 3, p. 21). This position strengthens the adrenal glands, kidneys and nerves, alleviates stress, and reinforces self-esteem and confidence. You are now likely to feel more calm and light-hearted.

Suggestion: The same hand positions can be used to treat someone else who is feeling rather fraught or lacking in self-confidence. If you are short of time, just do Steps 2 and 3. This will help you to gain strength, power and self-respect.

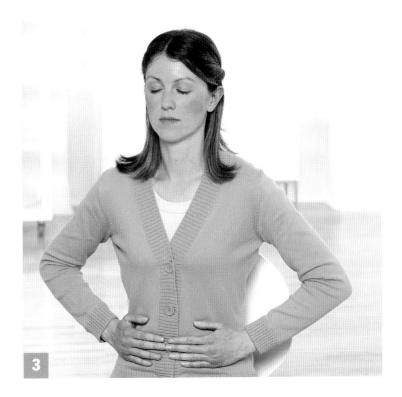

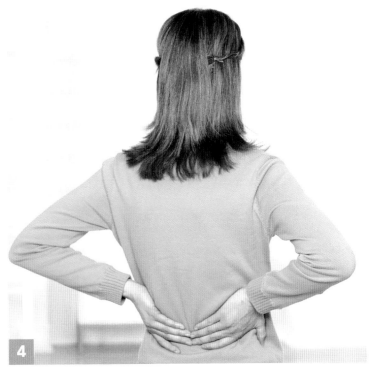

Job Interview Help

The Reiki Distant Healing technique – which is usually taught in the Second Degree – can be used to send positive thoughts and healing energy to a person, specific situation, theme or problem who or which is either far off in the distance or in the future. For example, you can use it to send positive energy to a situation you are going to be faced with yourself in the near future, such as an interview for a new job.

Second Degree practitioners use the Third Reiki Symbol (see p. 8) in order to transmit healing energy, as if "over a bridge of light" to the distant person or situation. The symbols and accompanying mantras work similarly to the vibrations of radio and television signals – invisible to the human eye. However, beginners to Reiki can also use a version of this technique without the symbols and mantras (see box below). Allow about fifteen minutes for the treatment and make sure you will remain undisturbed.

1 Close your eyes and cover them with your palms to connect with yourself. This position stimulates the third eye centre and enhances intuition and clarity of thought.

2 Now think of the situation to which you want to send healing – in this case your job interview scenario. Visualise it as specifically and positively as you can.

3 Give the situation a label or headline by finding one sentence to suit it, such as: "Job interview with (name of the interviewer and your own name) on (date), in (place)".

4 Raise both hands and draw the third Reiki symbol over the visualisation or its "headline". Then draw the first Reiki symbol on top of the third symbol to give the process more power. Say the mantras of both symbols three times, keeping your hands raised and allowing healing energy to flow out of both palms into the image.

5 Now imagine yourself in the job interview scenario. Visualise all the positive qualities you want to present: how you want to appear self-confident, relaxed, responsive to questions, intelligent, insightful and so on. After

> **Reiki beginners** *can practise Distant Healing simply by using visualisation and sending loving thoughts and positive energy to the desired situation via raised hands. The effect will not be as strong as for Second Degree practitioners, but it is still well worth doing.*

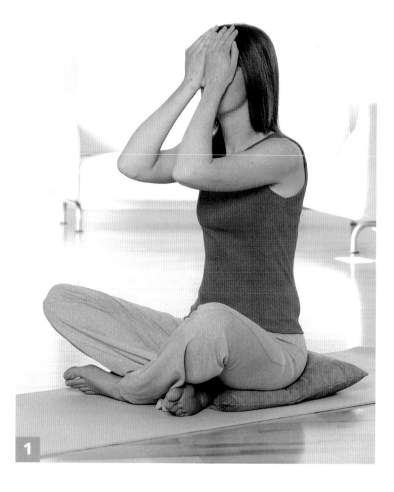

1

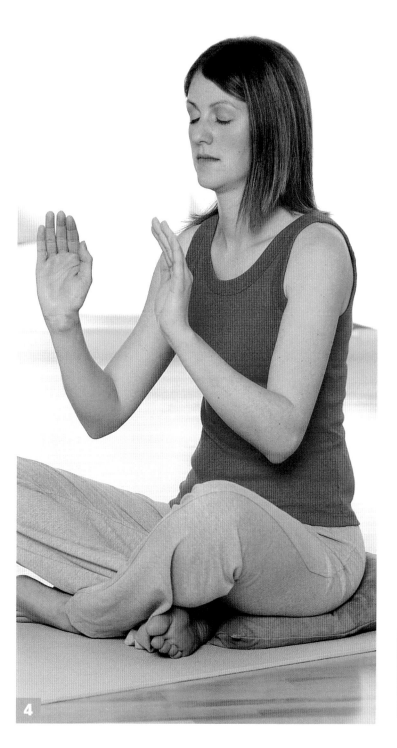

4

this visualisation, say: "For the highest good of everyone involved." This leaves it up to existence to determine whatever is the "highest good" for you and everyone else involved.

6 At the end you can visualise a colour around the whole situation, as if seeing it in a pink or gold balloon. Let go of the balloon image so that it can rise into the open sky. By letting go of the image, you can let go of the whole situation, accepting that you will get this job if you are meant to.

7 Finish your healing by thanking the Reiki healing energy for these blessings. Rub your hands to break the connection with the Reiki symbols.

CASE STUDY

Andrew had managed to secure a job interview but was aware that he often becomes nervous in pressurised situations and was worried that it might stop him from performing well. He asked a group of his friends to use Reiki Distant Healing on him and the situation, visualising him in a positive light and getting a positive outcome. Andrew later reported that he had never felt so calm and self-assured during an interview. In the end, he was offered the job.

Chapter 4

Free Time

"Let your best be for your friend. If he must know the ebb of your tide, let him know its flood also. For what is your friend that you should seek him with hours to kill? Seek him always with hours to live. … And in the sweetness of friendship let there be laughter, and sharing of pleasures. For in the dew of little things the heart finds its morning and is refreshed."

KAHLIL GIBRAN, *THE PROPHET*, 1923

FINDING – AND CREATING – TIME AND SPACE to relax your body, mind and emotions is essential in order to revitalise your energies and stay healthy. However, just "vegging out" and watching television every free evening or weekend is often not the best way to truly relax as it bombards your senses and imposes society's many expectations on you.

It is usually more emotionally nourishing and fulfilling to spend valuable time alone or with others, deepening your relationship with both yourselves and them. You might choose, for example, to start your weekend by taking an evening bath with calming oils to soothe your muscles and release any tensions in the body. You might then want to

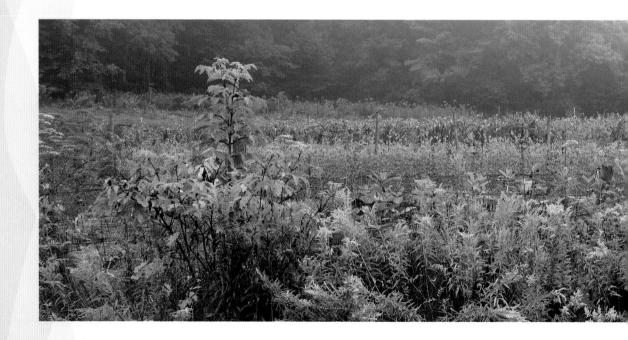

spend some of the rest of your weekend with good friends and family, playing in the park with your children or going for walks in the woods. Also make sure you leave some quality time to spend with yourself – doing anything from reading a good book to practising meditation.

It is also of great benefit to get enough moderate exercise during your free time, as this can release toxins in the body and set free any blocked energy caused by the build-up of life's tensions. Sometimes you need such physical activity to use up your energy before you can relax. For example, in the morning, before starting the day, you could do some stretching and yoga exercises to energise the body. Outdoor activities, such as jogging, cycling, hiking or just going for a long walk with a friend, are good ways to get physical exercise and also to gain the benefits of being out in nature, which can be particularly nourishing and soothing for the mind, body and soul.

Experimenting with how best to balance and spend your free time is all part of becoming aware of and sensitive to what you really need and what is good for you on all levels – physical, emotional and mental. Reiki can help you to develop this awareness of your own deepest needs and is an ideal way to take some time out for yourself and thus truly appreciate and value yourself. It is also an ideal way for you to enrich your friends' and family members' lives during their free time.

This chapter is divided into five sub-sections to help you decide which exercises or treatments might be most beneficial for you at any particular time – *Exercise and sport* (see pp. 82–3), *Connecting with yourself* (see pp. 84–7), *Connecting with friends* (see pp. 88–9), *Connecting with nature* (see pp. 90–1) and *Relaxation* (see pp. 92–5).

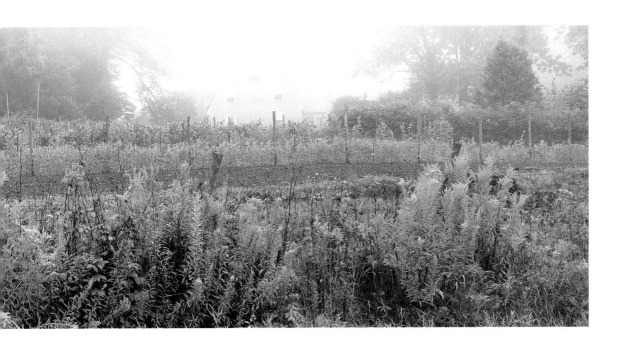

Exercise & sport

OUR MODERN LIFESTYLES and job circumstances often mean that we sit most of the day at a desk or in a car and do not get enough exercise to keep us healthy. This is a shame, given that the physical body – and especially the heart – love exercise and movement, and our bodies are built for movement. Every system in our body – from circulatory and lymph systems to muscles, bones and organs – perform best when we move and stretch regularly. To keep healthy and fit, therefore, we have to take care of this need for movement. The heart loves the vitality of beating and pumping, and the heart muscle can release all the body's tension if it gets enough exercise. Plus our breathing gets stronger as we take in more oxygen to help us get rid of toxins. In fact, researchers have found that moderate exercise stimulates the production of enzymes that help to protect the body's cells. Even little things – such as laughing, dancing or walking to town to do the shopping – support our energy to keep moving and keep us healthy. So, finding something active that we enjoy doing in our leisure time will soon bring obvious benefits.

Reiki is certainly not a substitute for physical exercise, sport or leisure. However, regular self-treatments (see pp. 18–21) may inspire us to get out and take part in something more active than just exercising the remote control from the comfort of our couch.

Reiki during Exercise: Self-treatment

You can also use Reiki to balance your energies and keep you energised during activities like jogging, hiking, yoga, stretching, aerobics, tennis and so on.

1 Whenever you feel exhausted during physical exercise, use Head Position 1, with the hands over your eyes, to centre you.

2 Then use Front Position 2 on the solar plexus to help re-energise you.

Suggestion: If you feel breathless while jogging, place your hands on the middle of the chest as you run in order to calm the energy in the chest and give support to the lungs.

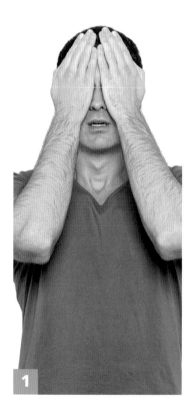

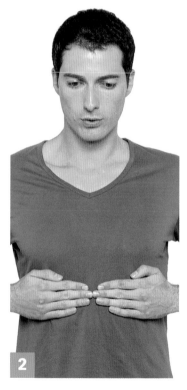

1

2

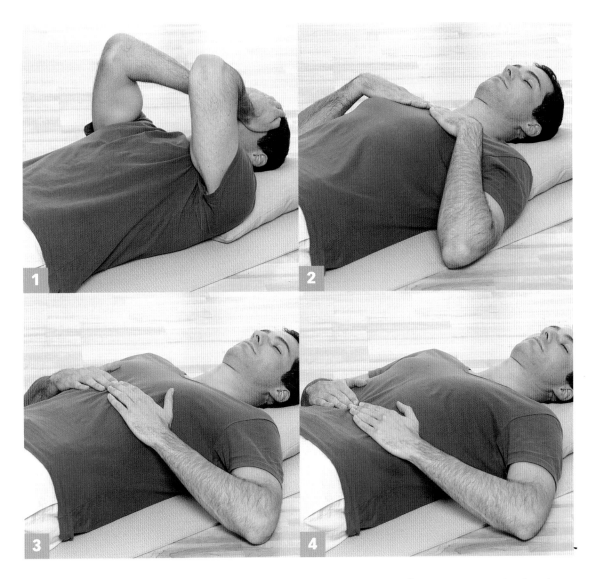

Reiki during Yoga: Self-treatment

Some yoga teachers include Reiki positions, and most students say that they feel a deeper relaxation between the yoga exercises as a result. Tapping into the Universal Life Energy during yoga also deepens the revitalising effect of the yoga practice. If you do yoga at home, try introducing some Reiki during the relaxation phase at the end, when you are already lying on your back.

1 Use Head Position 1, with your hands over your eyes, to relax you.

2 Use Front Position 1, with your hands on the chest, to strengthen the heart and lungs.

3 Use Front Position 2, hands on the solar plexus, to give you more power and strength.

4 Use Front Position 3, hands on the stomach, to help with your digestion.

Connecting with yourself

t is important that we use our free time to truly relax and restore our energy after the often frenetic pace of work and all of life's other pressures. Spending quality time giving Reiki to ourselves helps us to get to know ourselves and recognise what is best for us.

The fact that Reiki balances our energies means that we can use it to calm us down, let go of the week's events and reconnect with our true nature – our "inner being". By being in touch with this "inner being" we will intuitively know what is best for us in all areas of our lives. As long as we are open and willing to listen attentively, we will receive guidance from the source of our inner wisdom.

"Through the coming and going and the balance of life, The essential nature which illuminates existence is the Adorable One. May all beings perceive through subtle and meditative intellect The brilliance of enlightenment."

GAYATRI MANTRA TRANSLATION

Eleven Stages of Inner Healing – with Gayatri Mantra: Self-treatment

This self-treatment allows you to connect with and heal yourself on a deep level. It is best to keep your hands in each position for about five minutes, so allow about fifty minutes for the total treatment. You can play gentle, relaxing music in the background, if you wish. Alternatively, you could do a guided healing, where you have the chance to listen to the Gayatri Mantra (see p. 144).

The sound frequency of the ancient Gayatri Mantra – which is of unknown origin – is said to purify the atmosphere around us. When you listen to the mantra there may be a calming of the nervous system, and sincere practise of the mantra – either chanting or listening – can bring purification of thoughts and emotions and allow a feeling of inner peace and clarity to rise within.

1 Lie on your back, with your arms by your sides, breathing deeply.

2 Place your hands over your eyes, with your fingers together. Then say the following Gayatri Mantra several times out loud. Do not worry too much about perfect pronunciation of the Sanskrit, just remain full of positive intention:
*Ohm bhur bhuvah svah
tat savitur varenyam
bhargo devasya dhimahi
dhiyo yonah prachodayat.*

3 Once you have finished saying the mantra, place your hands in the middle of the chest and allow a feeling of peace to arise in your heart. Opening yourself to love and joy strengthens your heart and immune system.

4 Place your palms next to each other over your lower ribs and waist on the right side of the body. This helps to balances emotions such as anger and depression.

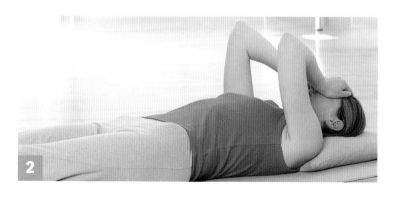

2

5 Then place the palms of both hands next to each other on the left side of your body to help digestive disorders and stabilise your immune system.

6 Now place one hand above the navel and the other below it. Relax into this area, allowing the healing energy to flow throughout your whole body.

7 Males and females should use slightly different hand positions for this step and the next:
Women rest one hand on each breast, tuning into the positive energy pole at the heart chakra.
Men place your hands in the middle of the chest and connect with the female energy inside.

8 Women place your hands in a V shape over the pubic bone and connect to the male energy inside (see p. 20).
Men place your hands wider, on each side of the groin, paying attention to the positive energy in the root chakra of the pelvic area (see p. 15).

9 Place your right hand over your forehead and your left hand below the navel, allowing a feeling of peace to spread from here into the whole body.

10 Cup your palms beneath your head, holding it like a ball and resting your hands on the cushion underneath. Let go of all thoughts and tension, so that your mind becomes soothed and calm.

11 Now let go of both hands and place them by your sides. Take a couple of moments to enjoy relaxing here. If you feel like it, wiggle your fingers and toes and stretch your body gently before slowly returning to a state of normal consciousness.

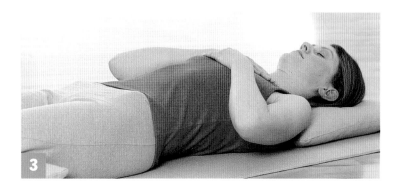

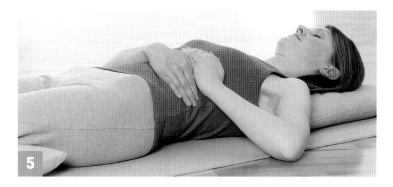

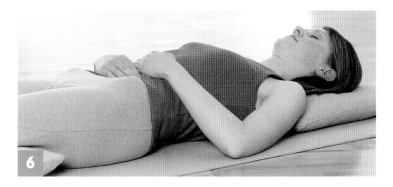

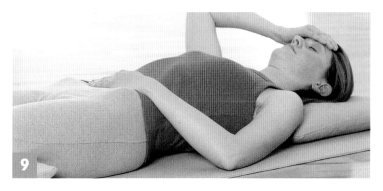

Whirling: Meditation

Whirling is one of the most ancient techniques used by the Sufi mystics. It involves you staying on one spot and moving your whole body around your centre. This technique will help you to get rid of tension, negativity and blocked energies in the body. You often see small children doing it naturally – just for fun.

It is always best to do the whirling exercise on an empty stomach. You can do it at the start of your day to restore and revitalise your energy. You may notice energy flowing like warm waves from the heart, down your arms and into your hands. Whirling before going to bed can also be beneficial: it helps you to have a good night's sleep by clearing any worries from your system.

1 Stand with your feet together, barefoot or wearing socks.

2 Hold both arms out at shoulder level, with your palms facing upwards. Alternatively, you can hold one arm up high, palm upwards, and the other arm lower, palm downwards. This way, your arms create a connection between heaven and earth.

3 Start rotating slowly – in whichever direction feels more comfortable – gradually building up more speed as you turn. Let your body be soft and keep your eyes open.

4 While whirling, look at one hand (the upper one if relevant) and focus on a particular finger to keep you from becoming dizzy. In the beginning, do

this for two or three minutes. Later, however, you may wish to increase the time to five, ten or even fifteen minutes.

5 When you want to stop the whirling, slow down the movement, cross your arms on your chest, and relax your head. This position helps to centre your energy so you do not feel dizzy. Stay like this for at least thirty seconds.

6 Once you have stopped, lie down on your front, close your eyes and feel your body melting into the surface beneath you. Stay here for between five and fifteen minutes; or if you do the whirling at night you might fall asleep this way.

Suggestion: Soothing music may help to relax you more into the whirling

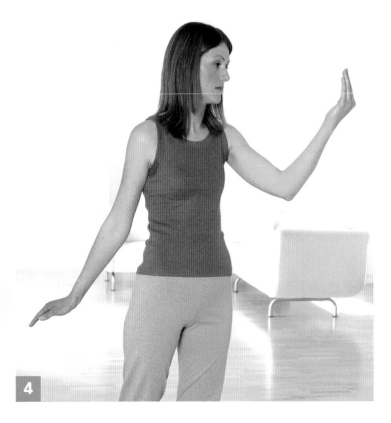

4

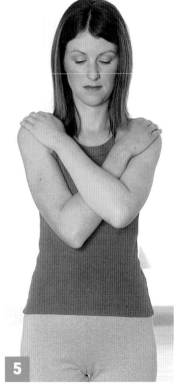

5

Laughter: Meditation

Laughter is the best medicine for the heart. It can change your body chemistry and affect your brain waves and your thinking. In addition, when you laugh, your breathing rhythm changes, which allows your heart and body to release tension. Laughing out loud also reconnects you with your inner child, making you feel young, vibrant and full of life and joy once more.

In some Zen monasteries, the monks start and end their day with laughter meditations. They believe it changes the quality of their day by allowing them to view situations less seriously. Having a good laugh at yourself and many of the situations you encounter creates space between you and your problems. Start looking out for situations and experiences in your day that can make you laugh.

This meditation will help you to laugh for no reason at all as soon as you wake up in the morning. You will gain most benefit if you do the exercise for five to ten minutes on a daily basis. Your eyes can be either open or closed.

1 When you wake up in the morning, start off by stretching your body.

2 After a minute or two, just start to laugh. In the beginning you will need to fake it: simply lift the corners of your mouth and laugh, even if you do not feel like it. Soon, however, your laughter will become real and spontaneous.

3 You can move your body to stimulate the laughing by throwing your legs up in the air or rolling around – whatever works and feels good for you.

Suggestion: You can do this meditation at any time of the day. If you do it with friends, you can trigger the laughter off by tickling each other or telling a joke, but remember not to get too involved in the external action. Instead, stay with your own laughter and use the other person just to stimulate the laughing in the beginning.

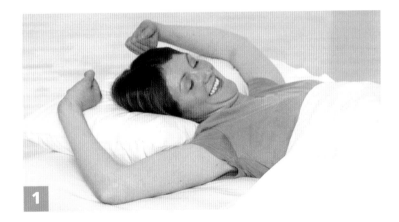

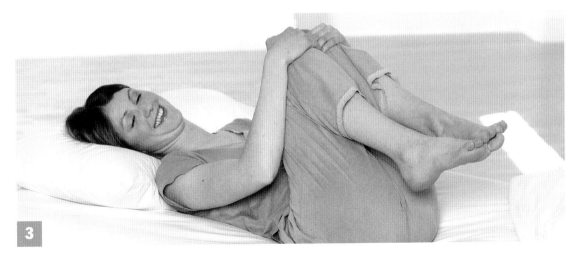

Connecting with friends

A LOT OF PEOPLE'S FREE TIME is spent with friends and family, so it is important to make this time emotionally fulfilling. After all, we don't just want to spend time with others, we want to spend quality time with them.

When we communicate by talking to each other, misunderstanding is always possible. Reiki, on the other hand, needs no words. It is a means of non-verbal communication that can create an intimacy between giver and receiver – a physical yet non-intrusive way to connect on a deeper level to another person. With Reiki, we tune into the other and follow our intuition about where to place our hands and how long for. Sharing Reiki among friends will enrich our relationships.

"Healing always happens from the heart – it is a loving and accepting space we share."

TANMAYA HONERVOGT

Reiki Sandwich

This treatment is performed in a group of three people. One person sits in the middle and is then treated simultaneously by the two givers sitting behind and in front of the central person. First, one of the givers smoothes the aura, stroking from the top of the head down to the floor. The hands of both givers are then placed intuitively on different areas of the body. To round off the session, smooth the aura once more. Then change over so that each person receives this Reiki treatment in turn. Spend about twenty minutes on each treatment.

Group Reiki

In a group treatment, the Reiki power flows more intensely. The receiver lies down and receives Reiki from all the rest of the group members. Groups can range from three to about seven people, with each individual receiving Reiki for about ten minutes on the front of their body and then ten minutes on the back.

It is a special experience to give and receive Reiki in a group of this size, as many hand positions are covered at the same time and the energy is much stronger. One giver can choose to focus on treating the knees and the soles of the feet, which have the reflexology points relating to the entire body and all its organs.

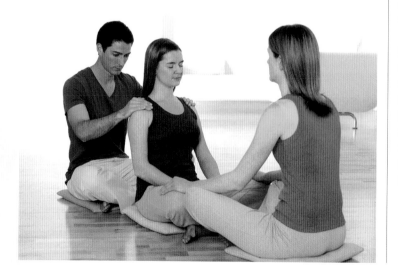

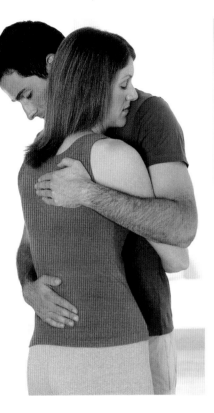

Giving & Receiving

This exercise is a way for you and someone close to you to share positive energy with one another in a non-verbal way. It can be a very nourishing and fulfilling experience. It is best to spend between five and ten minutes doing this exercise. You can play some relaxing music in the background if you wish.

1 Stand or sit in front of your partner with your eyes open, looking at each other with a soft gaze.

2 Hold your hands in front of you, with the right palm facing down and the left palm facing up. Then move your hands towards the other person so that you are gently touching one another's hands. Feel the energy connection between them, keeping your eyes open and looking softly at each other.

3 Imagine you are receiving energy from your partner into your heart chakra each time you breathe in, and you are giving energy to your partner from your solar plexus each time you breathe out. In this way you are creating an energy circle of giving and receiving between you. This can flow in a circular movement or in the shape of a flat figure of eight.

The Reiki Hug

A "Reiki hug" is a good way to thank someone else for giving you a Reiki treatment or simply to connect on a deeper level with a friend, as it is a nourishing way to exchange energy from heart to heart. Connect the upper bodies so that the left side of your chest is touching the left side of the other person's chest. This way, the energy can flow more freely. Stay as long as you like in this relaxed embrace. Your hands can rest on the other person's upper or lower back – whichever feels more comfortable for you both.

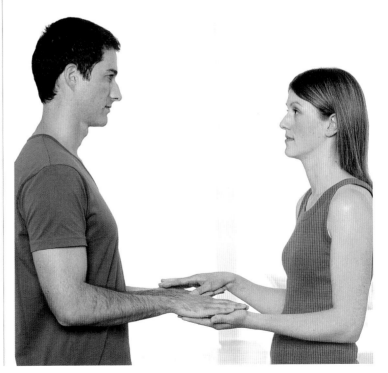

Connecting with Nature

SPENDING SOME OF YOUR FREE TIME OUTDOORS – whether relaxing in your garden, reading a good book in the local park, swimming in a lake, walking in the woods or hiking up a hill – will help you to connect with your earthly roots, to tune into your instincts, to connect with your intuitive and creative side and to become more in touch with who you really are at the core.

It can be immensely liberating to get away from all of the superficiality of the mechanical devices involved in so much of our daily lives and to be free of the physical restrictions of artificial walls. No external stresses or pressures; just enjoying the feeling of running free, breathing fresh air and living life fully in each moment, alongside Mother Nature.

Some Reiki exercises can be used to enhance this connection with nature and your connection with your true, inner self. Many other exercises are likely to increase your awareness of just how nourishing it is – for the mind, body and soul – to spend as much time as possible outdoors, being receptive to nature and feeling truly alive.

Connecting with a Tree: Exercise

When you are outdoors in a garden, park or forest, look out for a tree that you feel particularly drawn to – any one you want, for whatever reason you like. Each tree has a different vibration and sometimes you might feel attracted by the light, delicate energy of a birch, or the grounding, centring strength of an old oak tree. Doing this exercise will cleanse your chakras and revitalise your entire system.

1 Lean with your back against the tree. Then place one hand on your solar plexus and the other hand at the same height behind you, with the palm of your hand touching the tree. Close your eyes and tune into its energy.

2 Additionally, you can visualise drawing energy up from the earth, where the tree's roots are hidden in the ground. Imagine the energy entering your body through the soles of your feet as you breathe in. Let it flow up to the top of your head and higher, all the way up to the top of the tree.

3 When you breathe out, visualise the energy coming down from the tree, entering your body through the top of your head and flowing down your legs back into the earth.

Alternative

Instead of leaning your back against the tree, you can try leaning against the tree with the front side of your body. You can touch the bark of the tree with both palms, or place your arms around the whole tree, depending on its girth. Just choose a comfortable position and let yourself melt with the tree in this hugging position.

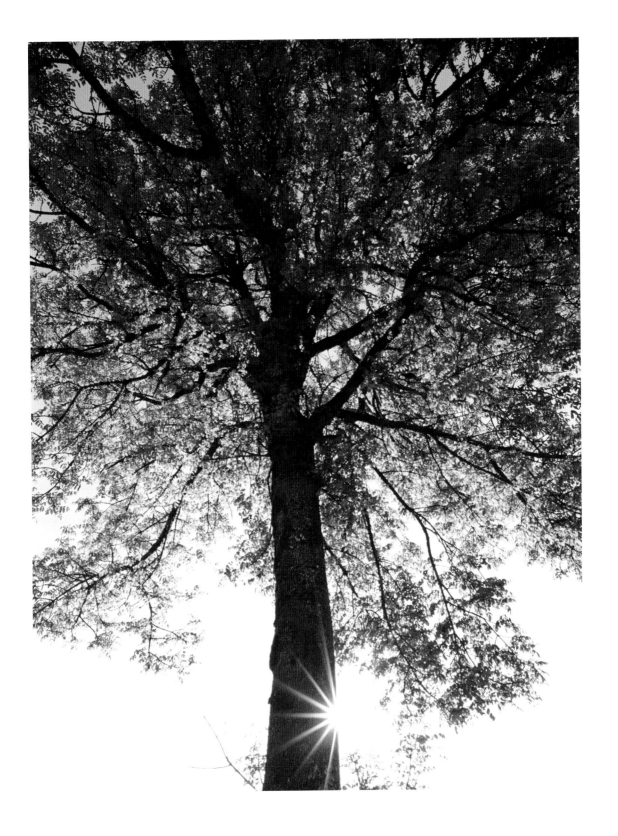

Relaxation

MANY PEOPLE FIND IT DIFFICULT to relax fully, which is a shame given its importance in helping us to stay happy and healthy. Relaxation cannot be forced. It happens by itself – like the bud of a flower opening. In moments of relaxation, you are simply there, resting in your own energy: the mind becomes still, and your thoughts – and therefore energy – are neither moving to the future nor to the past. It feels like that moment is enough; there is no asking for something to be different, no longing for something you do not already have. Relaxation is therefore a transformation of your energy from being goal-oriented to existing in the present moment. We often trick ourselves into believing that we will relax once we have achieved our goal. However, this kind of energy can dominate our life, as there is always something else that we feel we "must" achieve – thus, we never naturally "switch off" and relax. Relaxation techniques and meditation practices are therefore extremely useful as a means of introducing moments of valuable stillness into your life. Reiki is one such tool to help you to become more relaxed. The flow of Reiki energy relaxes the body and mind and, at the same time, refreshes and rejuvenates the whole body.

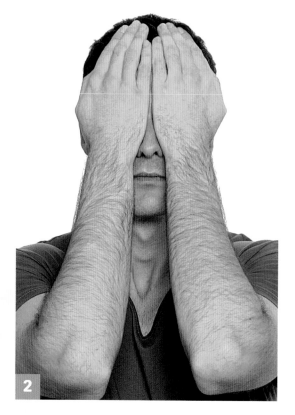

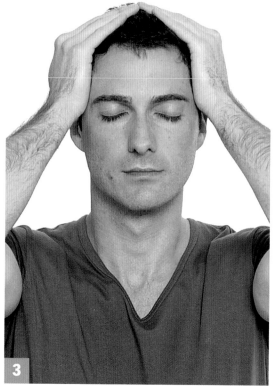

Enhancing Well-being: Self-treatment

Whenever you feel tense, tired or worried, take the time to relax and make a connection with yourself. This treatment will encourage you to feel nourished, peaceful and energised. Keep your hands in each position for between two and five minutes and so allow about twenty minutes for the total treatment. You can play gentle, relaxing music in the background if you wish. Alternatively, you could do a guided version of this healing (see p. 144).

1 Sit on a chair or lie down comfortably on your back, close your eyes and relax. Breathe deeply a few times and, while breathing out, allow your body to sink deeper into the surface beneath you.

2 Now place your hands over your eyes, resting your palms on your cheekbones, with the fingers close together. Relaxing your eyes relaxes the whole body.

3 Place your hands on both sides of your head, above your ears, with the heels of your palms touching the temples. This harmonises both sides of the brain, has a calming effect on the conscious mind and eases depression.

4 Now cup the back of your head with both of your hands, fingers pointing upwards. This helps to calm powerful emotions, such as fear, worry, anxiety and shock.

5 Lay your hands on each side of your upper chest, fingers touching just below the collarbone. This position encourages you to let go of negative feelings when you feel weak or depressed. It also increases your capacity for love and enjoyment of life.

6 To end your treatment, take a few moments to stretch your entire body gently, before slowly returning to normal consciousness.

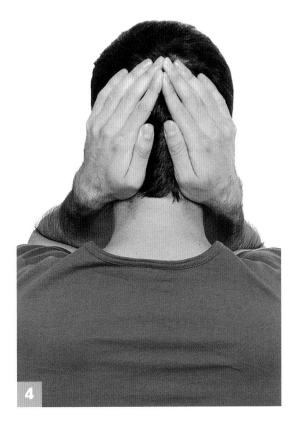

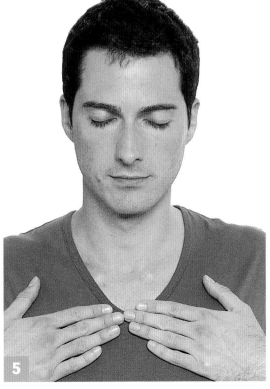

Reiki Before Sleep: Self-treatment

This treatment calms the body, mind and soul before you go to sleep, as well as harmonising all your chakras. If you happen to fall asleep during the treatment, don't worry – simply finish it the next morning. Keep your hands in each position for between three and five minutes. You can play gentle, relaxing music in the background if you like. Alternatively, you could do a guided version of this healing technique (see p. 144).

1 Place your hands over your eyes, resting your palms on your cheekbones. This connects you with your intuition.

2 Place both hands on the middle of your chest – the seat of your heart chakra. This strengthens your immune system and increases your capacity for love and the enjoyment of life.

3 Place one hand on your solar plexus and the other hand just below it – touching your stomach – allowing yourself to relax deeply into this area, and healing energy to flow throughout your whole body.

4 Place both hands in the shape of a V over your lower abdomen, with the fingertips touching over the pubic bone. This provides grounding and encourages you to trust more in life, which allows sleep to come more easily.

Suggestion: You can use this exercise effectively on yourself at any time you feel the need for an increased sense of calm and peace.

"During Reiki treatments I feel tremendously at ease and really enjoy the total relaxation."

LISA, 43, REIKI STUDENT

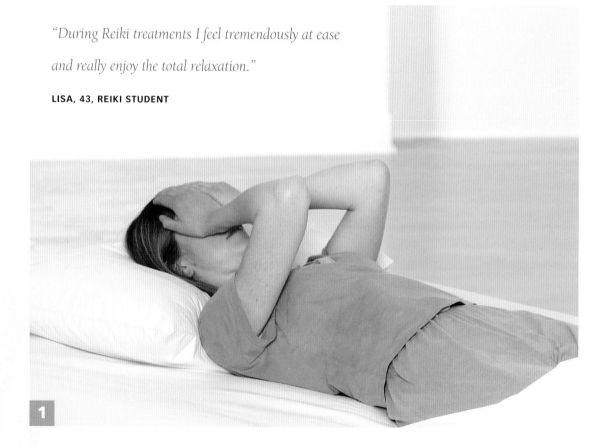

1

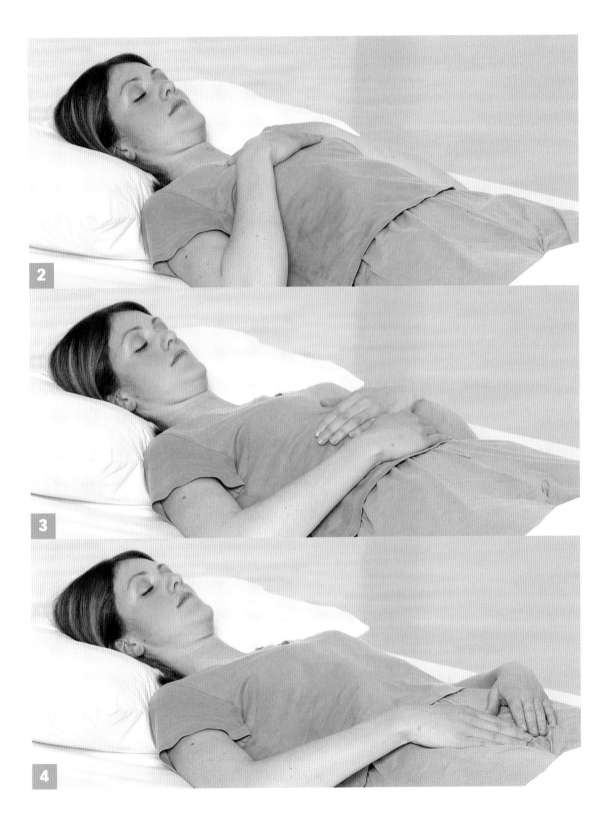

Chapter 5

Health & Well-being

"Could you keep your heart in wonder at the daily miracles of your life, your pain would not seem less wondrous than your joy. And you would accept the seasons of your heart, even as you have always accepted the seasons that pass over your fields. And you would watch with serenity through the winters of your grief. Much of your pain is self-chosen. It is the bitter potion by which the physician within you heals your sick self."

KAHLIL GIBRAN, *THE PROPHET*, 1923

UNDERSTANDING THE CONNECTIONS between illness, healing and health is one of the keys to health, happiness and harmony in life. Each person is a "whole", made up of body, mind and soul. The health of each "whole" person has two deeply interdependent aspects – the physical and the spiritual. The physical is the earthly, material part – the outer manifestation of the soul; the spiritual is the soul.

To be ill means that the body is no longer functioning as a whole: the harmony and balance have been lost. This kind of disturbance usually takes place in the mind first and is only later manifested as a physical symptom. As every illness is trying to give us a specific message, it is crucial that we recognise and accept this message. If we can sense it at the start, an imbalance is unlikely to reach the physical sphere. If, however, we do not listen to and understand such initial messages, the body tries to find a more direct and visible language, in the form of discomfort or pain. For example, when we feel obliged to go to a social event but would have preferred a quiet evening at home, or when we force ourselves to go into work when we are feeling really run down, the body might well find its

own way for us to take some time off by catching a cold or getting a headache or migraine. In serious cases, the body might even form an ulcer or succumb to a heart attack. So we must listen to the body's subtle signals.

We need to love, respect and take care of our body in order to stay both physically and emotionally healthy. If we neglect it, we will not be able to find inner harmony and well-being. We also have to develop a feeling for and an awareness of our body, and ourselves, so that we can recognise our real needs. In today's society we live so much "in the head" that we are often cut off from our bodily feelings, yet the body and its instinctive feelings reconnect us with our source of energy and are often what make us feel truly alive. When we are alive, and full of joy and energy, any physical complaints are much less likely to take root and develop into full-blown illnesses.

Reiki works on all levels – physical, mental, emotional and spiritual – in the prevention and the treatment of all sorts of illness. Reiki rejuvenates our energy, which is normally used up in daily activities, and strengthens our immune system. Reiki can help with many conditions – both acute

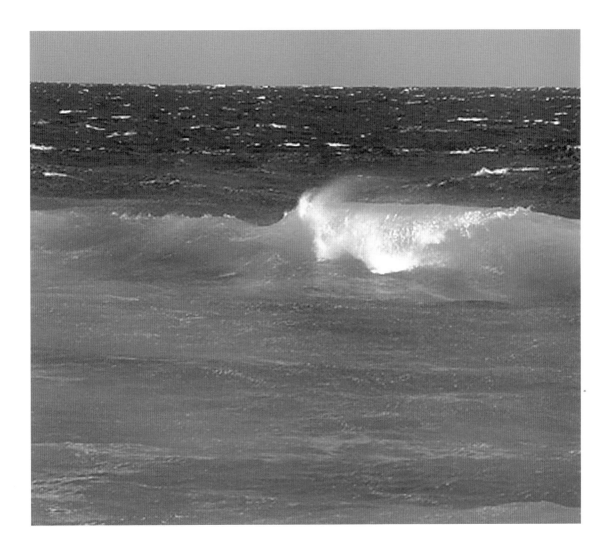

and chronic – and can be given in conjunction with any other treatment. Many complementary therapists use it to supplement and intensify their work, whether acupuncture, chiropractic, massage, homeopathy, cranio-sacral therapy, aromatherapy or reflexology. Reiki can also enhance traditional medical treatments as it cleanses the body of toxins and supports the body's ability to heal itself.

People are sometimes subconsciously attached to illness. Although, on a conscious level, they want to be rid of the disorder, the illness can subconsciously become part of their identity, which makes them reluctant to let go of it. Reiki treatments can make sufferers aware of the underlying causes of their pain and thus help them to transform negative patterns into positive, healing ones.

This chapter is divided into sections that relate to five of the key factors in maintaining both physical and emotional well-being: *Healthy eating* (see pp. 98–9), *Supporting the energy of the heart* (see pp. 100–103), *Dealing with illness* (see pp. 104–111), *Acceptance* (see pp. 112–13) and *Calm* (see pp. 114–17). These headings should help you to find which Reiki treatments and exercises are most suitable for you or your friends and family at any given time.

Healthy eating

MANY PEOPLE IN TODAY'S HECTIC WORLD are suffering from dietary imbalances. The fast food, sugary drinks, sweets, white bread, French fries, milk products, red meat and canned food being consumed simply do not give us the balanced supply of nutrients our bodies need to stay healthy. When imbalance occurs the first signs we often encounter are low energy, poor digestion, aches and pains, excess weight and foggy thinking. If ignored, however, these can soon turn into more serious health problems.

Researchers have found that eating healthy food and getting the best nutrients help to avoid many problems in the first place. Even serious health challenges, such as diabetes, cancer and heart disease, can, in certain cases, be directly linked to diet. A good diet, along with moderate exercise, is therefore not only the key to keeping an ideal body weight, but also to overall health and well-being.

Reiki develops our intuition and helps us to become more in touch with what our body really needs and doesn't need – in dietary terms – in order to stay or become healthy. It is also a means for us to send positive energy to the food we eat, making it even more nutritious – for the soul as well as for the body. We need to take responsibility for our own health and make the necessary dietary changes if we want to stay fit and healthy.

Fasting with Reiki

Fasting is an ancient method of physical detoxification that allows the physical body to feel freer and lighter. When done in combination with meditation, it also enhances purification on a spiritual level. Fasting usually involves a limited intake of certain foods over a period of several days.

Fasting can help to treat various disorders but should always be done under the guidance of a nutritional expert. Seek the advice of your doctor if you have any serious medical condition.

Reiki is an effective support for fasting as it mitigates unpleasant side effects by speeding up the elimination of toxins that has been set in motion. Since the Reiki energy fortifies the immune system, which is not being "fed" as much as usual, it is a good idea to give yourself a full-body treatment (see pp. 18–21) every day during a fasting period.

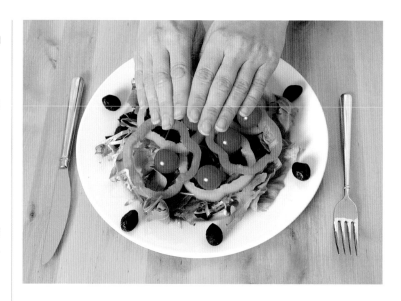

Energising your Food

You can enrich, cleanse and energise the food you eat quite simply by holding your hands over or around the items to be eaten for between 30 and 60 seconds and sending out positive energy. Second Degree practitioners can take this process a step further by drawing the First Reiki symbol – taught in the Second Degree – above the food. The Reiki power thus released helps to increase the nutritional value of your food by charging it with positive energy and intention.

Eating Disorders: Self-treatment

The underlying reason for many eating disturbances, such as anorexia and bulimia, is often emotional. If possible, it is a good idea to give sufferers of such disorders a full Reiki treatment every day (see pp. 12–17) in order to develop their inner strength and deepen their sense of security and self-confidence. Or, if you recognise that you suffer from any dietary problems yourself, give yourself the gift of a daily self-treatment (see pp. 18–21). Either way, it is recommended that you spend extra time on the hand positions shown on the right.

You can also use the Reiki Mental Healing technique (see p. 24) to try to discover the true reasons behind your eating disorder.

1 Use Head Position 2 (see p. 18).

2 Use Head Position 4 (see p. 19).

3 Use Front Position 3, with hands either side of the navel (see p. 20).

4 Use Back Position 3, with hands over the kidneys (see p. 21).

"Reiki helped me to find myself again, to get back in touch with my true self."

BETTINA, 30, TEACHER

CASE STUDY

Susan was in therapy because she tended to use food as a substitute to cope with the stress of her job. Whenever she felt low in self-confidence, she started eating too much. After only four Reiki treatments, she was already starting to feel calmer and more in touch with her body. She now feels more able to recognise her own needs and sense what is and isn't good for her. Reiki integrated something for her and as a result she feels physically healthier and mentally clearer.

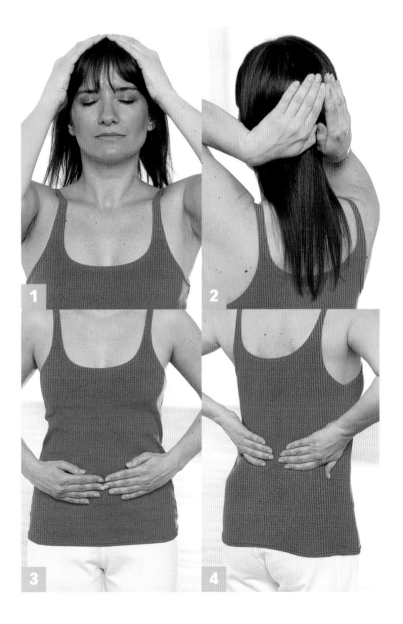

Supporting the energy of the heart

Today, many people find themselves living a way of life that means they are excessively busy all of the time and constantly under pressure – at work and at home. As a consequence of this, they feel restless and impatient with themselves as well as those around them. This set of circumstances often burdens our entire physical health, but especially the heart.

Contrary to the popularly held belief, it is the heart and not the head that is our primary source of wisdom and understanding. the heart contains a vast space in which we can find spontaneous peace, love and joy at any time, without any particular reason.

When the heart can relax and beat in its own rhythm, it is the healthiest and most content. The more you know yourself and are in touch with your heart, the more you are able to look at the events in your life in a calm and peaceful way. And when you see all the challenges and experiences of life as a gift, you will find the inner strength and courage to act from a peaceful and accepting space in any situation, which will greatly enrich your whole life.

Relaxing the Heart through Sighing: Self-treatment

This very simple but effective exercise helps you to release any blockages and tensions from the heart. It is particularly useful when you find yourself worrying or feeling stuck with a certain emotion that you cannot seem to let go. This is because the act of sighing is a wonderfully easy way to take the pressure off your heart and to release worries, fears or anything else you are hanging on to. The negative energy frees itself as you breathe out.

1 Take a deep breath in and allow your jaw to relax as you breathe out through an open mouth, making a deep sighing sound. Repeat this a few times, relaxing completely with each out-breath.

2 While sighing, place your hands over your eyes to help you to reconnect with yourself.

3 Additionally, visualise any event, thought or feeling from the past that you are still hanging on to and that is preoccupying your mind, and invite it to leave you with the out-breath. Just breathe it out on a mental level.

4 Now place both hands on the chest. Pay close attention to your heart and notice if you feel any different – any lighter or freer, for example.

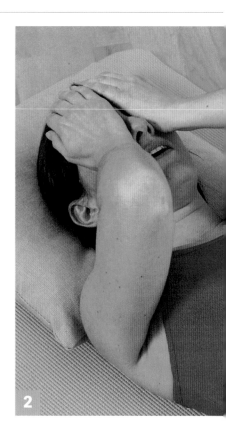

Talking to your Heart: Self-treatment

This exercise helps you to reconnect with your innermost feelings and it is a good way to release the day's worries and tensions before gong to bed. The heart intuitively knows your needs and you can ask it about anything that burdens you or to which you need a solution. Just talking to it, like to an old and trusted friend, can be a deeply healing experience.

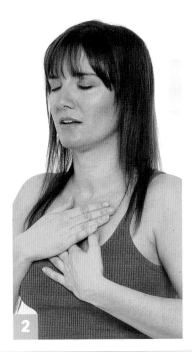

1 Sit or lie comfortably in silence, become still and give Reiki to your eyes. While doing this, concentrate your attention on your heart. If you sense a heaviness or constriction in the heart, try sighing to gain relief.

2 Connect further with your heart by placing both hands on the middle of your chest, where the heart centre (fourth chakra) is located.

3 Now start talking to your heart as if it were an old friend. Ask it questions, if you like, such as "How are you?" and "Can I do anything for you?", and wait to receive answers from within.

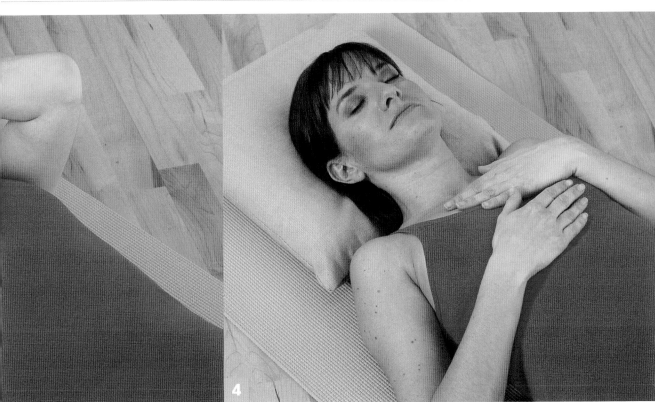

Heart-protection Exercise: Self-treatment

Chinese medicine is based on a system of what are called meridians. These are energy lines that provide the organs, and indeed the whole body, with vital energy. Chinese healing arts, such as acupuncture and acupressure, involve stimulating various points along these meridians in order to activate the energy of certain organs or body systems. For example, if you have problems with your heart – whether physical, emotional or both – you can use the pressure points called "Shenmen" and "Shaochong" on the heart meridian, to release any tension in that area.

Acupuncture point: "Shenmen"

1 Raise your left hand in front of you, palm facing inwards, and place the thumb of your right hand on the little finger side of your left wrist – just below the base of the palm, where there is a small indentation. Then apply a little pressure to this spot.

2 Stretch your left hand towards your body and back to the neutral position, keeping the right thumb in place. Do this movement between ten and fifteen times. You might feel a little tingling – this is a healthy sign indicating that the blocked energy is shifting.

3 Then repeat the whole process on the other hand. Treating these points relaxes the heart meridian and shifts blocked energy along it, so that the heartbeat can become regular again.

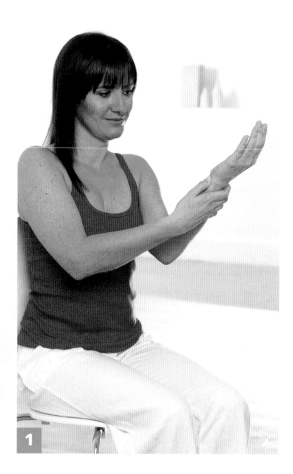

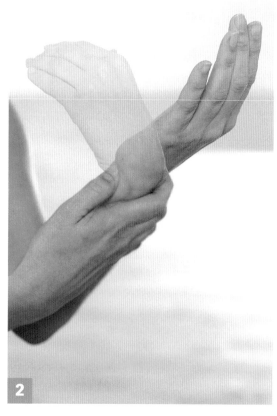

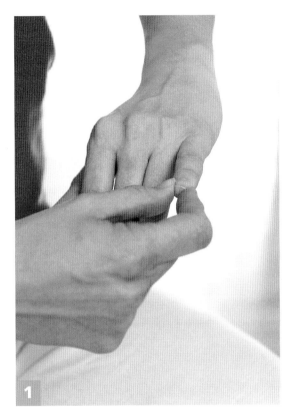

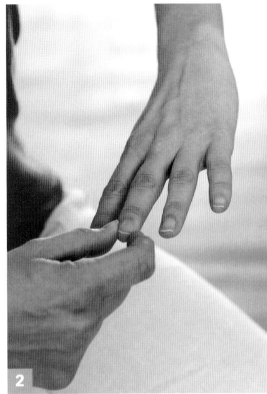

Acupuncture point: "Shaochong"

1 Hold the little finger of your left hand – palm facing down – with the index finger and thumb of your right hand, and turn and press it for a while as strongly as you can. The pressure point here – on the bottom outside corner of the little finger nail – is the end point of the whole heart meridian, which begins at the armpit. Stimulating it nourishes and balances the energy of your heart, so if you feel considerable discomfort or even a little pain while pressing, it is an indication that there is a blockage in the energy.

2 Now apply pressure to the same points on all your other fingertips in order to stimulate and balance your whole body's energy. The tip of your middle finger is connected to your pericardium – the tissue surrounding the heart – so applying pressure to this point supports your heart's function.

3 Then repeat the whole process to the fingers of the right hand. If you turn and press your fingers in this way every day, you will notice after a while that it no longer feels uncomfortable, indicating that the energy is now flowing more smoothly through the meridians. If you don't have time to treat all the fingers, just treat the little and middle fingers.

Suggestion: If ever your doctor needs to take a sample of your blood, it is worth asking for it not to be taken from the middle finger – according to Chinese medicine, this can weaken the heart.

Dealing with illness

REIKI CAN HELP to treat both chronic and acute disorders by strengthening the body, as well as stabilising the immune system and, in many cases, lessening the pain. It is recommended to start with a daily treatment for a minimum of four days to allow the healing energy to build up and, therefore, speed up the healing process.

Start by talking with the receiver about their symptoms and explaining that the Reiki healing energy adjusts itself to the needs of the recipient. Make them aware that self-healing reactions, such as an urgency to go to the bathroom, hunger or thirst, chilliness, warmth, a headache or even increased pain initially, may occur after the first sessions. These are a necessary part of the healing process, in which the body's "toxic energy" has to reach a certain peak before being able to leave the body. Some receivers may also have a strong emotional reaction. This is the body releasing blocked energy and suppressed emotions. Simply continue the treatments normally until a sense of balance is restored. A minimum of six to twelve sessions is recommended.

In cases of extreme pain, it is advisable to give short Reiki treatments at frequent intervals to the affected area of the body – for example, twice a day for twenty minutes. When giving Reiki after shocks and injuries, such as broken bones and burns, be aware that the pain may initially worsen before beginning to subside.

Treating Tinnitus

Nowadays our senses are often overloaded with multiple stimuli. Technology is developing so quickly that we are not yet fully aware of all the long-term effects that the gadgets we use, such as cell phones, may have on the human body. More and more young people have problems with their ears and suffer from tinnitus, an unpleasant disorder traditionally associated with old age. Tinnitus sufferers experience an almost constant ringing sound in their ears, which can vary from mild to extremely loud, like the drone of a plane engine, in the worst cases. Twice-daily practice of this short treatment can bring great relief. Stay in each hand position for between five and ten minutes.

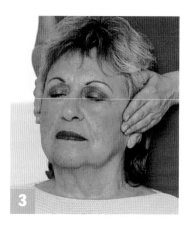 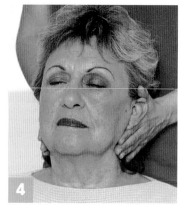

1 Use Head Position 3 (see p. 19).

2 Use Front Position 1 (see p. 20).

3 Treat the ears directly by placing the little finger of each hand in the entrance of each ear.

4 Place your palms behind the receiver's ears, with the thumbs above and slightly in front of the ears.

Suggestion: If you have more time, you could integrate this selection of hand positions into a full-body treatment (see pp. 12–17).

Pain in the Shoulders and Arms

As well as relieving pain in the shoulders and arms, this treatment can help with general bone complaints and boost circulation. It is best to stay in each hand position for about five minutes, which means that total treatment time is between twenty and thirty minutes.

1 Ask the receiver to lie down on their stomach, turning the head to one side.

2 Place your hands next to each other on the receiver's right upper shoulder, the base of your palms touching the spine and your fingertips touching the shoulder muscle.

3 Place your palms next to each other on the left shoulder in the same way, this time keeping the base of your palms on the shoulder muscle and the fingertips pointing towards the spine.

4 Ask the receiver to turn and lie on their back. Place your hands on the top curve of each shoulder, fingertips pointing downwards so that they are touching the receiver's upper arms.

Suggestions: When there is pain in the lower arm, keep one hand on the shoulder area and place the other at the elbow. When there is pain in the hands, keep one hand on the shoulder area and place the other at the wrist.

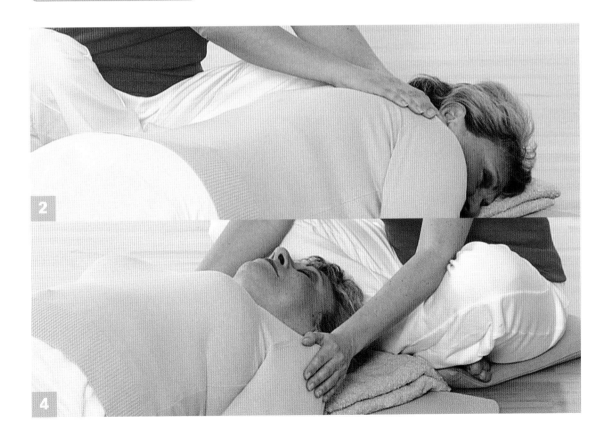

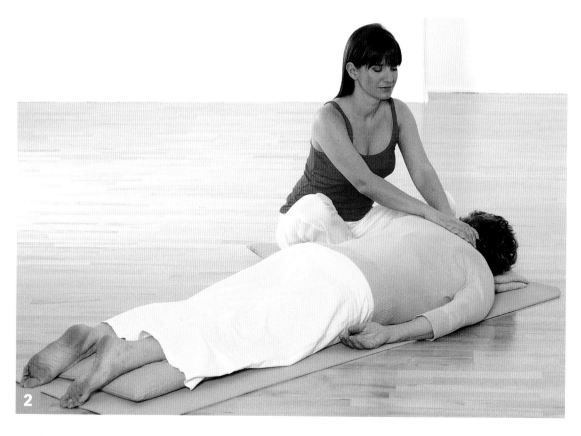

Neck & Back Pain

This treatment is excellent to use when you have a painful back or neck, such as after a whiplash injury, and is also good for generally "sore bones" and for growing pains. The emotional causes for pain in the upper back and neck can include holding back emotions or feeling overloaded with responsibility. The middle back holds repressed feelings, such as guilt, worry and not being open to receive. And pain in the lower back is often associated with a lack of emotional support in life, a lack of abundance, and difficulties with sexual expression. It is best to stay in each hand position for three to five minutes, which means you will need about thirty minutes for the total treatment session.

1 Ask the receiver to lie down comfortably on their stomach.

2 Lay one hand on the nape of the neck and the other on the top neck vertebra.

3 Place your palms next to each other on the left shoulder, with the base of the palms on the shoulder muscle and the fingers pointing towards the spine.

4 Move your hands onto the right upper shoulder, this time with the base of the palms on the spine and the fingers pointing to the shoulder muscle.

5 Now repeat Steps 3 and 4, starting with your hands almost one hand-width further down the back each time, until you have covered the whole back.

6 Lay one hand horizontally across the sacrum and the other at right angles to it, over the coccyx – to form a T. This allows the energy to travel up the spine.

7 Finally, keep one hand covering the coccyx and place the other hand on top of the neck. Keep both hands in this position until the flow of energy feels the same in both hands.

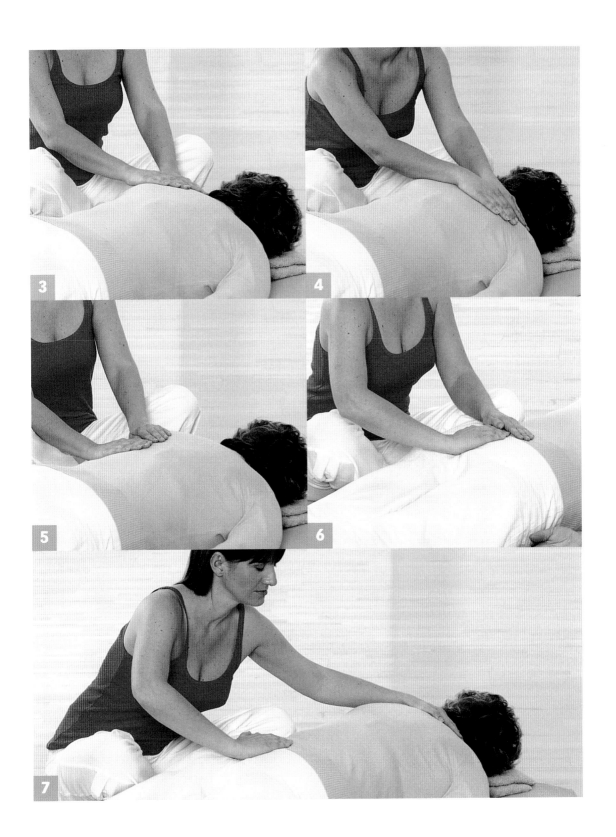

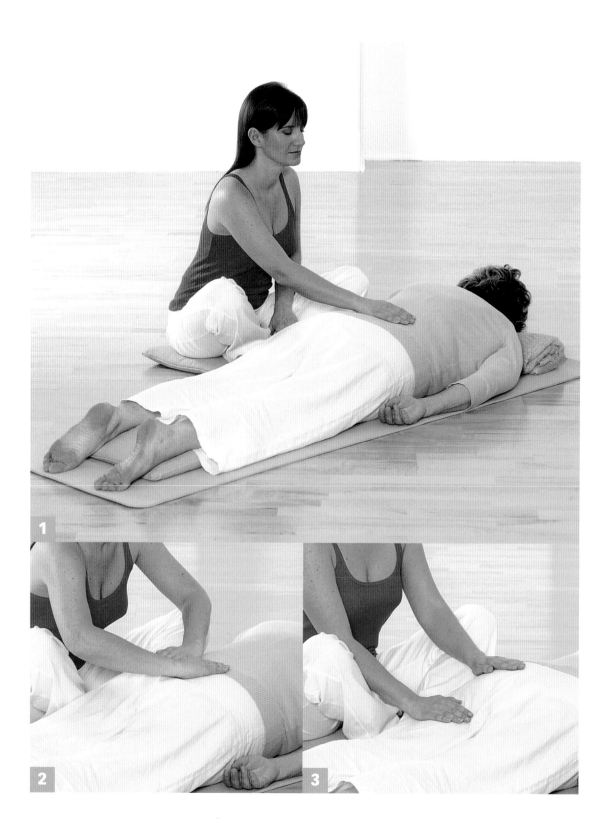

1

2

3

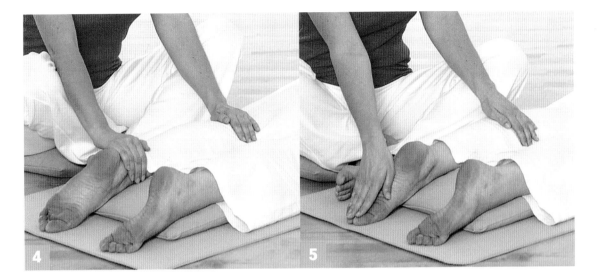

Sciatic Pain

The sciatic nerve starts at waist level on both sides of the spine and runs down through the buttocks and legs. Sciatica generally occurs when some point along this nerve becomes trapped by surrounding muscles. It can cause great pain and is sometimes accompanied by a tingling or numbness in the legs. However, emotional factors, such as holding back emotions or not feeling supported in life, can also contribute to its occurrence.

It is particularly effective to treat sciatica with Reiki in conjunction with chiropractic treatment, but Reiki on its own can also considerably lessen the pain. Stay in each hand position for three to five minutes, so that your total treatment time should be twenty to thirty minutes.

1 Ask the person to lie down on their front and then gently place one hand at waist level on their spine.

2 Place one hand over the sacral bone, with the fingertips pointing downwards, and the other hand beside it, with the fingertips pointing upwards.

3 Lay one hand directly on the buttock of the more painful side, or over the sacrum, and move the other hand – one hand-width at a time – down the leg on the same side, until you reach the knee.

4 Keep one hand on the knee and, with the other hand, work your way down the leg – one hand-width at a time – to the heel.

5 Place one hand on the sole of the foot and the other hand just below the knee.

6 Then treat the leg on the less painful side in the same way, in order to balance the body's energies.

CASE STUDY

Yvonne, aged 34, had a slipped disc, a two-year-old injury to her lower back and sciatica, including numbness in her right leg. After receiving Reiki the stiffness and pain in her leg disappeared. With each treatment, she experienced more sensation returning to her leg, and she felt more refreshed and energised.

Detoxification and Digestive Disorders

This treatment helps with any detoxification, digestive and metabolic problems by treating the kidneys, adrenal glands, liver, gallbladder and the digestive organs, such as the duodenum, spleen, pancreas, stomach and intestines. It also balances emotions, such as anger, depression, fear, or shock, arising out of emergencies and accidents. Keep your hands in each position for about five minutes. Total treatment time required should, therefore, be between forty and fifty minutes.

1 Ask the receiver to lie down comfortably on their back. Use a pillow or cushion under the head, knees and/or lower back if needed.

2 Ask the receiver to close their eyes and take three or four deep breaths, sighing with each out-breath to let go of any tension in the body. Meanwhile hold both the feet and tune into their breathing rhythm.

3 Next, move to one side of the receiver and smooth the aura by moving both your hands in a stroking action – above the body – from the head down to the feet. Repeat this three times in total as it has a relaxing effect on the receiver.

4 Now lay your hands in Front Position 2 (see p. 14), one hand on the lower right ribs and the other directly below it at waist level. This is helpful for hepatitis, gallstones and metabolic disorders.

5 Next, use Front Position 3 (see p. 14) on the left lower ribs and waist. This is helpful for diabetes, infections, anaemia and leukemia. It also helps stabilise the immune system in AIDS and cancer patients.

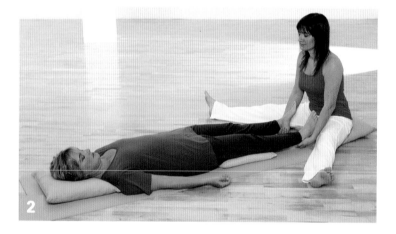

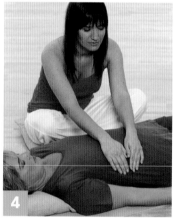

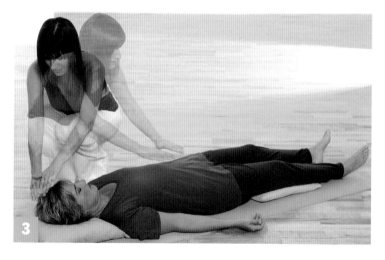

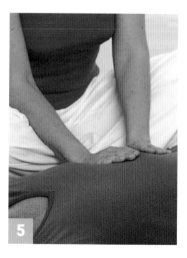

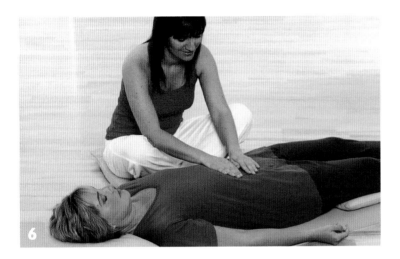

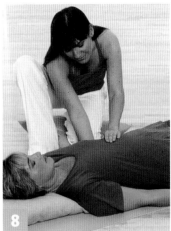

6 Place your hands in Front Position 4 (see p. 15), one hand above and the other below the navel. This treats intestinal disorders, nausea, indigestion and bloated feelings.

7 Now, move round to the receiver's right side and place your left hand underneath the right side of their back, at waist level – where the kidneys are located. At the same time, place your right hand over the lower front of the ribcage. This helps to balance the kidneys, which is particularly effective for the treatment of allergies, such as hay fever, as well as for back pain.

8 Move back to the left side of the body and this time place your right hand under the left side of the back and your left hand over the lower front ribcage – at the same level as before.

9 Now place your left hand over the spleen area, on the lower left side of the ribcage, and lay your right hand across the thymus gland, which is below the collarbone. This position stimulates the immune system and helps auto-immune disorders.

10 Use Front Position 1 – the T Position (see p. 14) – for fortification of the immune and lymphatic systems.

11 End the treatment by stroking the receiver's aura again – twice in a downward direction and once from the feet to the top of the head. The last upwards stroke can be repeated, as it helps the person to come back to normal consciousness more easily.

Suggestion: Playing soothing music in the background often helps the receiver to relax more easily.

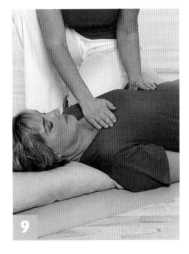

"An ill person is one who has simply developed blocks between himself and the whole, so something is disconnected."

OSHO

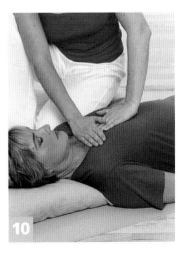

Acceptance

ACCEPTANCE ARISES OUT OF A DEEP TRUST towards life. When we accept events as they come, no matter what happens, we liberate ourselves from the restrictions of our own likes and dislikes. It is usually easy for us to accept and welcome the pleasurable events in life, but it is not so easy to accept the unpleasant ones. After all, it is human nature to fight pain. However, developing an ability to accept both emotional and physical pain allows us to start learning from all the experiences we live through.

When we learn to look at the events that occur in our life as an opportunity for inner growth, then we cease to be a victim. We take responsibility for everything happening and can see that since we have – at least in

some way – created our own situation, we also have the power to change it if we wish. For example, when we experience serious illness, pain or the death of a loved one, we may feel depressed, helpless and unable to understand "why on earth" this is happening to us. However, it is essential to surrender to a higher will and trust that this higher force knows the divine plan of our life and that it is for the best in the end.

Reiki can help you to develop this ability to accept – firstly, by making you more aware of the pain underlying your feelings of anger, frustration, helplessness and hopelessness, and, secondly, by helping you to balance and transform these emotions.

Dealing with Feelings of Helplessness: Self-treatment

When you go through periods of feeling completely helpless in life, it can be very beneficial to give yourself a full Reiki treatment every day (see pp. 18–21), spending extra time on Head Positions 2, 4 and 5. Front Position 3 is also important, as it balances and energises the solar plexus (the power chakra), as is Back Position 3, which calms the adrenal glands and supports kidney function.

Pinpointing Pain: Self-treatment

We can look at pain – whether physical or psychological – as part of our growth process in life. Whenever something hurts us, we need to acknowledge the feeling and move further into it rather than trying to repress it. All wounds need exposing before they can heal.

This exercise really helps you to focus on and accept your pain. It is best to try this technique first with physical pain, such as a headache or stomach cramps, before trying it with emotional pain, such as feelings of abandonment or of loneliness.

1 Sit silently and focus your whole mind on the pain and intensify the feeling.

2 Pinpoint exactly where the pain is, and try to "listen" to it and concentrate on it further.

3 Become watchful and notice the pain start to shrink. If you do not see a change, try to visualise the pain shrinking in your mind's eye, allowing it to come to a sharp point, like that of a needle. Then just remain with it.

4 Notice what happens to the sensation of pain. It may well lessen or even disappear completely as you simply observe and accept it.

Dealing with Frustration: Self-treatment

Feelings of frustration are an indication that we have had some kind of expectations that have not been met. This exercise will help you to let go of the initial expectations and, in turn, the feelings of disappointment.

1 First, lay your hands directly on the place where you feel the emotion most strongly, whether in your heart, head, chest, back, solar plexus or wherever it might happen to be.

2 Use Head Position 1 (see p. 18).

3 Use Head Position 2 (see p. 18)

4 Use Head Position 4 (see p. 19).

5 Balance the energy between the heart and throat by placing one hand on the heart chakra – on the middle of the chest – and the other gently around the throat. This encourages you to express anything you are frustrated about.

Suggestion: In cases of extreme or ongoing frustration, it is better to give yourself a full Reiki treatment (see pp. 18–21). It can also be useful – before giving Reiki to yourself – to find some quiet place where you can act out repressed emotions by beating a cushion or screaming out loud.

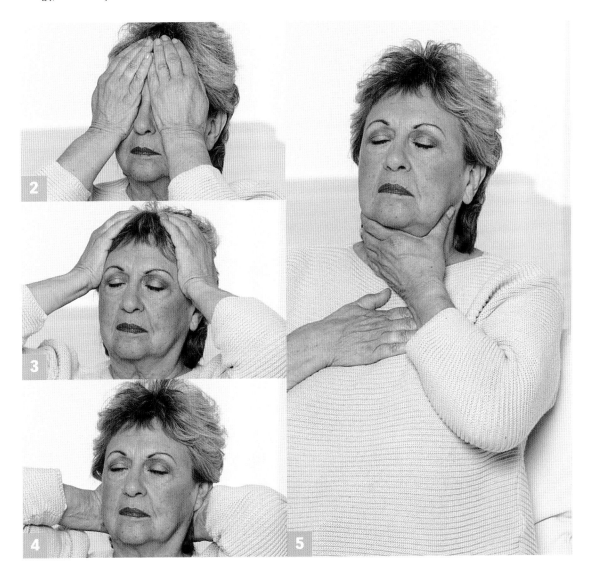

Calm

WE TEND TO EVALUATE EVERYTHING that happens in life and label it as either "good" or "bad": we either like it or don't like it. However, if we can instead take a wider view of the events in our life, we can become more aware of the cycles of life itself, which are neither good nor bad. They simply belong to the process of life, like the different seasons in nature, and the wonders of birth and death; and they all offer a challenge for us to grow and to discover who we really are.

We tend to underestimate the power of our mental forces and ignore the fact that our thoughts can create our reality for us. If we are in a negative mood and have negative thoughts, we therefore create a negative reality in that moment, which invites negative feelings – such as worries, fears, depression, guilt, anger and so on.

The Universal Life Energy, called Reiki, transforms these negative feelings, which have lower frequencies, into positive feelings, which have higher frequencies. In this way, Reiki acts just like love – the most healing force there is, which heals not only the body, but also the mind and the soul. Reiki can, therefore, help us to learn to love and trust ourselves, and to relax more deeply and thoroughly, connecting us with the core of our being and making us more calm and still.

When you Feel Fearful: Self-treatment

This Reiki treatment will help you to let go of any fear you may be experiencing, encouraging you to connect with feelings of trust and joy. It will also strengthen your nervous system and relax the adrenal glands. Remain in each position for a minimum of five minutes, making a treatment time of about forty minutes in total. It can also be useful to lay your hands directly on the place where you or the other person feels the fear most strongly.

1 Use Head Position 1 (see p. 18).

2 Use Head Position 4 (see p. 19).

3 Use Front Position 1, over the chest (see p. 20).

4 Use Front Position 3, either side of your navel (see p. 20).

5 Use Back Position 3, over your kidneys (see p. 21).

6 Place one hand on your forehead and the other hand on the back of the head.

7 Keep one hand on the forehead and lay the other hand on the solar plexus.

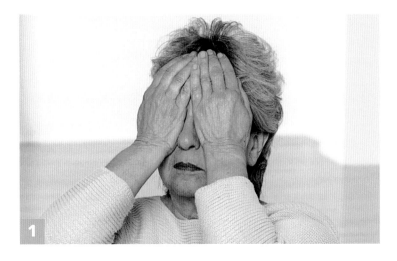

1

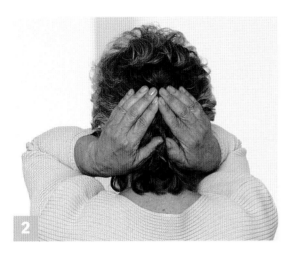

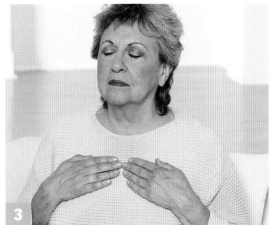

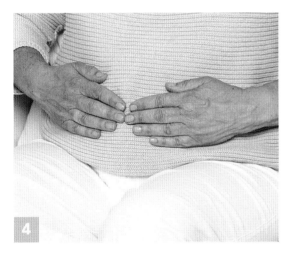

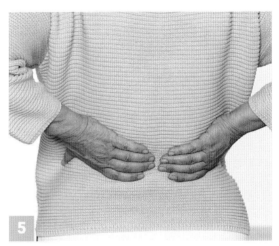

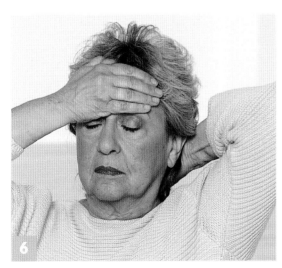

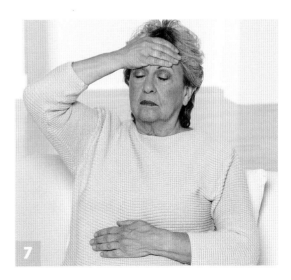

When you Worry: Self-treatment

If you tend to worry excessively, give yourself a full Reiki treatment every day (see pp. 18–21). This will strengthen your confidence and self-esteem. However, this is the ideal short sequence to allay your worries if you do not have time for a complete treatment.

1 Head Position 1 (see p. 18).

2 Head Position 2 (see p. 18).

3 Front Position 1, on the chest (see p. 20).

4 Back Position 3, over the kidneys (see p. 21).

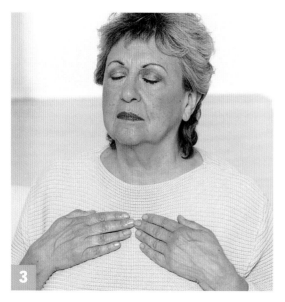

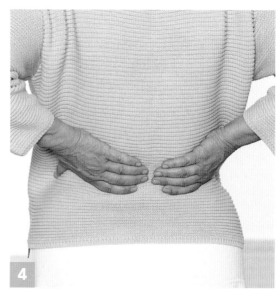

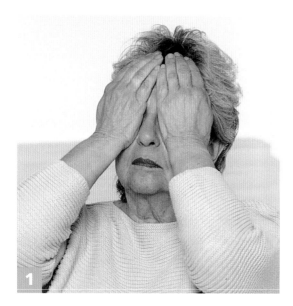

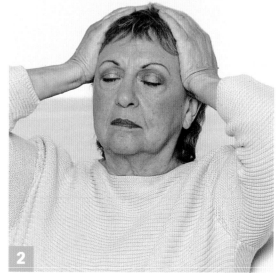

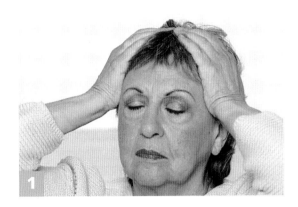

"If I am facing a problem I ask for guidance from the Universe and Reiki. For me, Reiki is the best medicine, it heals everything."

ANNE, 25, REIKI STUDENT

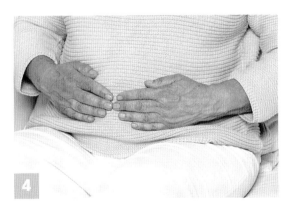

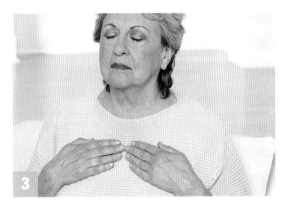

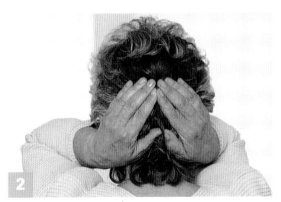

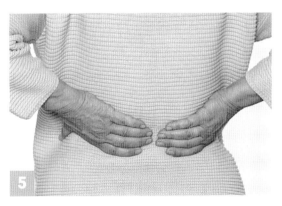

When you Feel Depressed: Self-treatment

This treatment helps ease symptoms of depression by increasing the production of endorphins – the body's "happiness hormones" – and promoting a feeling of self-esteem and inner power (see pp. 18–21 for a further explanation).

1 Use Head Position 2 (see p. 18)

2 Use Head Position 4 (see p. 19).

3 Lay your hands in Front Position 1, over the chest (see p. 20).

4 Move your hands to Front Position 3, at either side of the navel (see p. 20).

5 Place your hands in Back Position 3, over the kidneys (see p. 21).

Chapter 6

Life Stages

"Some of you say, 'Joy is greater than sorrow' and others say, 'Nay, sorrow is the greater'. But I say unto you, they are inseparable. Together they come, and when one sits alone with you at your board, remember that the other is asleep upon your bed. Verily you are suspended like scales between your sorrow and your joy. Only when you are empty are you at standstill and balanced."

KAHLIL GIBRAN, *THE PROPHET*, 1923

LIFE IS A CONTINUAL MOVEMENT from birth to death: the moment we are born we are already growing older. It is natural, then, that everything is continually changing throughout our life. We experience many "deaths" and "rebirths" – for example, when we first leave our family to live on our own, when we give birth to our first child, when we are going through difficult life phases such as puberty, the menopause or a midlife crisis, when we separate from a partner, when our children eventually leave home or when a loved one dies … Nothing is certain in life and material objects have no lasting substance.

All the losses and changes we experience in life offer us valuable opportunities to grow and to train ourselves to let go of old habits, patterns and thought processes. When there is an unexpected event in life, such as being made redundant, losing a life partner, or a sudden change of house or living standards, we often react negatively. But these negative emotions are almost like toxins in the body, and if we don't deal with them creatively, they can cause a "dis-ease". We need, therefore, to become aware of the negative feelings and transform them into positive ones – of understanding, patience, tolerance, flexibility and

forgiveness – in order to heal our relationships with both ourselves and others. Reiki can help this process by healing the areas that require the most attention – on physical, emotional, mental and spiritual levels – thus transforming our responses to suffering.

The key factor in maintaining emotional balance and health throughout all life's challenging stages is learning how to relax into the present moment, without resisting and constantly struggling against the fact that things change. There are many moments in life when we can practise letting go of objects, events or people gracefully, becoming detached from them and relaxing into our true nature. The pains of life and love are all stepping stones for our own growth towards liberation from suffering.

However, if we have a "should" lurking anywhere in our minds in terms of this detachment – for example, that we "should" not be affected negatively by events – the all we do is build up layers of denial and repression. Only our willingness to experience the pain and sorrow, as well as the joy, that comes with our experiences provides the ground for us to realise that which can never be lost – the true, innermost essence of our own being. Experiences

come and go but our divine essence is permanent. To truly know who we are – call it consciousness, light, God or truth – leads to liberation from suffering, confusion, negativity and fear (see also "Self-recognition", p. 36).

This chapter is divided into eight sections that offer guidance through the most challenging phases we tend to face in life: *Adolescence* (see pp. 120–1), *Pregnancy* (see pp. 122–3), *Separation* (see pp. 124–5), *Menopause* (see pp. 126–9), *Midlife crisis* (see pp. 130–3), *Empty-nest syndrome* (see pp. 134–5), *Bereavement* (see pp. 136–7) and *Transition* (see pp. 138–9). The last of these sections helps us to confront the reality of our own mortality.

Adolescence

ADOLESCENCE IS THE PERIOD OF TRANSITION during which we are suspended between childhood and adulthood. It is a difficult time as both the body and the psyche go through significant changes. During this time, we have to let go of our childhood and find the strength and courage to define our own individual stance on life. It is as if we are stepping into a new identity: our interests change from games and toys to relationships and sexuality. This can be a very isolating time and can bring much uncertainty about our new roles in life. Teenagers also quite often suffer from a lack of confidence about their physical appearance. They feel helpless as their own body undergoes such dramatic changes in a relatively short period of time.

Adolescent years are also characterised by a great desire for freedom and self-determination, as teenagers become aware that all sorts of new possibilities lie ahead to be explored. This can cause rifts to emerge in relations with parents, as teenagers often feel a need to rebel against them or close themselves off emotionally from them.

Reiki can help teenagers significantly during puberty by increasing their sense of self-trust and self-security, lessening feelings of isolation, and easing problems such as growing pains (see *Neck & Back Pain,* p. 106), mood swings and acne. It can also support hormonal changes, aid detoxification of the body and promote relaxation in the midst of all the upheaval and uncertainty.

Treating Acne

The skin problem known as acne most often appears on the face, upper back and shoulders. It is common among teenagers, as it is often related to an upsurge of hormonal activity, but it can also be the result of over-acidic blood caused by consuming excessive amounts of refined food, dairy products and foods high in fat and sugar, such as chocolate and fizzy drinks (see also *Healthy Eating*, pp. 98–9). Acne is often worse if anger, fear or other strong emotions are being held in, as whatever is not expressed may cause the skin to erupt. Giving this Reiki treatment to a teenager may well help their acne disperse, as well as help to boost their self-confidence. Keep your hands in each position for at least five minutes.

1 Use Head Position 1 (see p. 12) as it helps allergies and balances the pineal and pituitary glands, which govern the hormones in the body.

2 Use Front Position 1 (see p. 14) as it treats the thymus gland and strengthens the immune system, helping to rid the body of the toxins that can cause acne.

3 Use Front Positions 2 and 3 (see p. 14), as this treats the liver and gallbladder, aiding detoxification.
4 Use Front Position 5 (see p. 15) to treat the reproductive organs. Note that it is not necessary to touch this area if the receiver is uncomfortable with it. You can, instead, keep your hands a little above the body.

5 Lay your hands on the kidney region, as in Back Position 3 (see p. 16), to help with allergies and to detoxify the body.

Suggestion: When working over inflamed areas on the skin, it is a good idea to place a sterile gauze pad on the sensitive area before laying on your hands.

Teenage Angst & Suppressed Emotions

Giving this treatment to a teenager will help them to let go of strong emotions and negative feelings. The positions involved help to strengthen the nervous system and relax the adrenal glands. Keep your hands in each position for a minimum of five minutes.

1 Lay your hands in Head Positions 1, 2 and 4 (see pp. 12–13). These calm your mind and emotions and stimulate an increase in the production of endorphins, which can be thought of as the body's "happiness hormones".

2 Lay your hands in Front Position 1 (see p. 14). This helps you to let go of negative feelings and connects you with your heart, increasing the capacity for love and the enjoyment of life.

3 Lay your hands in Front Positions 2 and 3 (see p. 14) to ease powerful emotions, such as fear and frustration, and to help to increase self-confidence.

4 Lay your hands in Back Position 3 (see p. 16), over the kidney area. This relaxes and strengthens the nerves, and reinforces self-esteem and confidence.

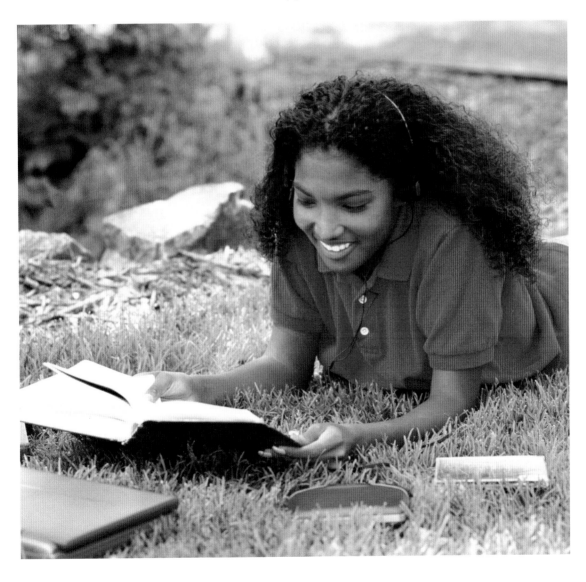

Pregnancy

PREGNANCY IS A VERY SPECIAL and precious time. What a gift it is for a woman to be able to carry life in her own body and to deliver a new human being into the world. As well as comforting and reassuring the developing child, Reiki during pregnancy can help the future mother by helping her to connect more deeply with the living being inside her. Receiving Reiki in early pregnancy can also help to ease the discomforts of the hormonal and physical changes that take place in the body and, in later pregnancy, can ease any worries about the actual birthing process.

If you are a future mother or father, it is rewarding to simply place your hands on the mother's belly as often as possible to deepen the connection between you and your baby. Some future parents are moved to tears by the wonder of this experience. You can also talk to the baby in the womb, either silently or out loud.

> **CASE STUDY**
> *Catherine was giving her pregnant friend a Reiki treatment when she felt that the baby had become very quiet and turned his head in the direction of the energy. The friend, who was in the fifth month of her pregnancy, enjoyed it very much and, apparently, the baby did, too.*

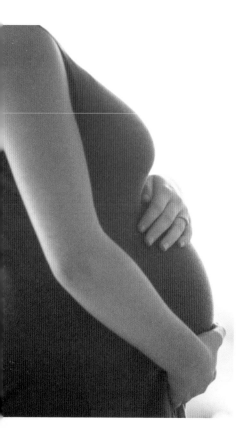

During Pregnancy: Self-treatment

In early pregnancy you can give yourself a full Reiki treatment (see pp. 18–21) or be given a full treatment by someone else (see pp. 12–17), spending most time on the areas requested by the receiver.

This treatment, however, is suitable throughout pregnancy and is usually so relaxing and calming that any worries, concerns or fears about possible complications regarding the birth simply fade away.

1 Give Reiki directly to areas in the belly where you most sense the baby.

2 Place your hands on your heart area, in the middle of your chest, to intensify the feeling of union between you and your baby.

3 Then place your hands on your lower back to ease any pain you might have been experiencing.

Suggestion: When giving Reiki to a woman in the advanced stage of pregnancy, it is best not to give Reiki for much longer than half an hour, concentrating mainly on the areas where she is feeling any discomfort.

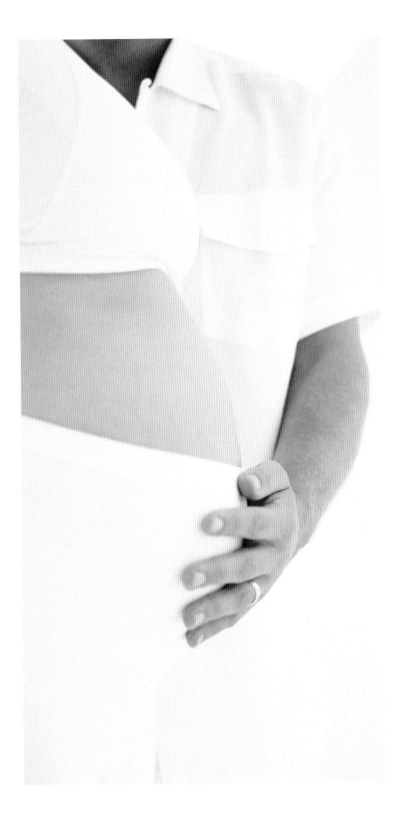

Distant Healing to the Birthing Process

The Distant Healing technique – usually taught only in Second Degree Reiki – can be used to send healing to the birthing process of someone close to you, even if you do not know exactly when labour is likely to begin. However, you should always ask the permission of the receiver before you do this.

Draw the Distant Healing symbol once in the air in front of you, followed by the First Reiki symbol directly behind it to increase the healing power. Repeat the mantra for each symbol three times and then say the name of the pregnant woman and a description of the situation she is in three times.

Suggestion: You can also send distant healing to yourself, in advance, for the birth of your own baby. Visualise the Reiki "switching on" when labour begins, until about two hours after.

> **Reiki beginners** *should hold their hands out in front of them, visualise the pregnant receiver, say their name out loud and direct healing energy and loving thoughts towards them.*

> **CASE STUDY**
> *Mary gave a Reiki session to a friend in the last stages of her pregnancy. She enjoyed it hugely; became very relaxed and let go of any fear about giving birth. Shortly afterwards she gave birth to a healthy baby girl and felt that the Reiki had helped her remain more at ease about the birthing process.*

Separation

The end of a relationship or dissolution of a marriage usually brings immense change and uncertainty to life. All our anxiety, dissatisfaction and regrets about our inability to make the relationship work confront us with strong emotions. We can be disturbed by feelings of abandonment, bitterness, anger, guilt, sorrow, pain and fear of the future. However, these deep experiences of suffering and loss can also encourage us to take the first step on the path towards spiritual growth.

Reiki can help us to move positively through this time of change, bringing a clarity to the mind and helping us to make good decisions. It also helps to calm excess mental activities, such as the invented dialogues that we often play and replay in our own minds. Reiki also supports us in finding deeper meaning in painful circumstances and in making the changes in attitude and lifestyle that are necessary to promote a happier and healthier life.

Reiki cannot necessarily help us to avoid a separation, but it can give support during the process, helping us to separate in a loving way. To be able to let go of the other person, we need to let go of any blame and anger we might still hold. We need to forgive the other person for what they have done and ask them for forgiveness when we have wronged them. Reiki's Universal Life Energy can help us to transform negative feelings into a willingness to connect with our partner's beauty, love and uniqueness.

Reiki During Separation: Self-treatment

If a separation is unavoidable, Reiki will provide support for you in your sorrow and grief. It is a good idea to be kind and loving towards yourself by implementing a full self-treatment (see pp. 18–21) every day. However, if you are lacking in time, try the short treatment below instead.

1 Use Front Position 1 (see p. 20) to support your capacity to forgive.

2 Use Front Position 3 (see p. 20) to ease powerful emotions.

3 Use Head Position 1 (see p. 18) to give clarity of thought and intuition.

4 Use Head Position 4 (see p. 19) to release fear and further emotions.

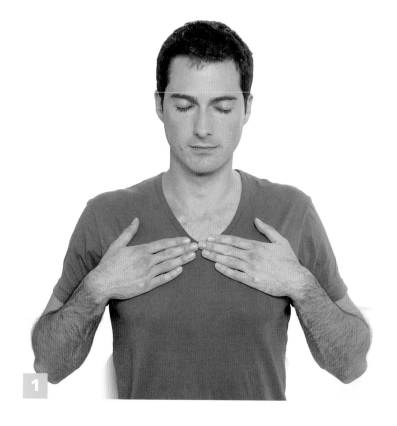

1

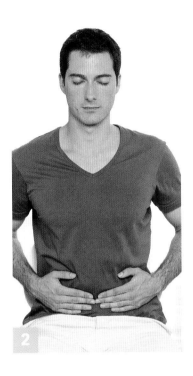

" Reiki helped me to travel down a new road by providing energy and fresh insight, and helping me to let go of old, less healthy ways of being."

SAM, 35, REIKI STUDENT

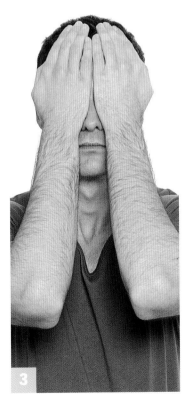

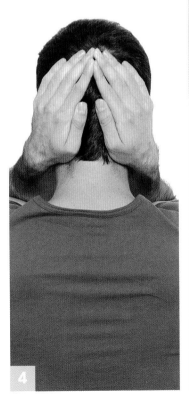

Psychic Protection: Self-treatment

The rose is a universal symbol for love and is mentioned as a symbol for psychic protection in many esoteric writings. The visualisation of a rose can be used as protection against the negativity and projections of others. The use of this visualisation is supposed to leave your heart open towards the other person, but not allow it to be affected by their negative energy. It can also enable you to gain greater awareness of maintaining your own space and identity yet be fully present with the other person. It is therefore particularly useful when you are going through a separation, as it is difficult enough to deal with your own mixed thoughts and emotions without being constantly affected and weighed down by your partner/ex-partner's emotions and projections, too.

1 Visualise a rose halfway between you and your partner/ex-partner whenever you do not want your energies mixing. Alternatively, visualise a rose on the edge of that person's aura. You can also do the visualisations during a phone conversation.

Suggestion: "The rose of protection" can also be used each night before sleep. Visualise it in front of you, with all the events of your day inside it, and allow the image to dissolve.

Menopause

THE MENOPAUSE is also called "the change", which is a good indicator of the many life changes that occur at this time. Strictly speaking, menopause is the cessation of the menstrual cycle and the capacity to bear a child in women. It is a transition that most often happens in a woman's mid-forties to fifties, when her hormone balance begins to shift. Some of the symptoms encountered are hot flushes, night sweats, mood swings, vaginal dryness, disturbed sleep patterns and lapses in memory. Increased fat levels in the blood can also result from menopausal changes, and some women fear the loss of sexual enjoyment and worry about osteoporosis. This phase in life can therefore be accompanied not only by physical problems, but also by spiritual and emotional problems.

Researchers have now found that some middle-aged men, too, can suffer from menopausal symptoms similar to those experienced by women. Reduced levels of testosterone – the male hormone – cause this.

Medical doctors tend to prescribe hormone-replacement therapy (HRT) for women who are having problems during this time. These treatments, with supplemental oestrogen and progesterone, may reduce some symptoms, but they can mean a higher risk of unwanted fat, water retention and even cancer. A German gynaecologist, Dr Volker Rimkus, has found that it is also beneficial for men and women in middle age to take certain natural hormones that have an identical chemical structure to the body's own hormones.

Nowadays, there are many more alternative ways to treat menopausal symptoms. Natural herbal remedies such as wild yam, agnus castus, black cohosh and isoflavones made from soya beans, work as hormonal balancers in that they contain natural oestrogen and progesterone, and support the natural hormonal system.

Some people may also benefit from other complementary treatments such as homeopathy, Chinese herbal treatments, Bach flower therapy and Reiki healing.

Women in some Eastern and developing countries appear to make the menopausal transition without many problems. This may have a lot to do with cultural diet, as the traditional foods of native peoples in countries such as the USA, Mexico and Papua New Guinea include, for example, wild yam; and soya products are a big part of people's daily diet in Asian countries. In some native cultures, the menopause is seen as a cause for celebration – a time when a woman reaches the peak of her womanhood. She has completed the circle of childbearing years, is entering a new level of self-discovery and is looked up to as a "wise woman" in the community.

Menopause in Western society, on the other hand, can be an emotionally charged time, especially if we are in denial about the ageing process. Reiki, however, can help us look at this new phase of life in a positive way, as one that gives us the opportunity to revise outgrown attitudes, drop old habits that have become an obstacle, and let go of unhealthy addictions or a lifestyle that no longer suits us. It encourages us to take a fresh look at ourselves, to find our own solutions to problems and to set our priorities differently, affirming the mature, wise woman inside by finding our deeper purpose for living.

To help the body in this time of change, it is useful to keep to a healthy diet – low in fat and high in fibre – as this will help the body adjust more easily to changing hormonal levels. It is better to eat less meat, sugar and refined foods, and more fresh fish, fruit and vegetables. It is also beneficial to take suitable nutritional supplements and to stretch and exercise regularly.

Treating Menopausal Symptoms

Reiki can help women during the menopause on all levels – physical, emotional, mental and spiritual. On the physical level, it will assist in balancing the endocrine system, which influences the production of hormones in the body. On the emotional level, Reiki can harmonise reactions to any unpleasant physical symptoms. On the mental level, Reiki connects us with intuition, inner strength and courage. And spiritually, Reiki will allow more space to adjust and to accept that we are entering a new phase in life. The Reiki Mental Healing Technique (see p. 24) – taught in the Second Degree – is particularly beneficial.

" I experienced a very deep sense of calm and peace. I felt that I had entered a very special place within me and felt certain that Reiki was a very welcome addition to my understanding of life."

MICHELLE, 52, REIKI STUDENT

Treating the Reproductive Organs

This Reiki treatment can be used to treat either male or female reproductive organs to ease any discomfort in this area, as well as help with disorders of the bladder or urinary tract. If you do not like direct body contact in these areas, ask the giver to keep their hands a little above the body.

1 Use Front Position 5, placing your hands in the shape of a V over the pubic bone. The hands should touch at the bottom if treating a female but should be wider on the groin when treating a male (see pp. 15 and 20).

2 Place your hands beside each other on the right side of the lower abdomen, with your hands in such a way that the outside of the lower hand touches the pubic bone.

3 Then place both hands next to each other at the same height on the left side of the lower abdomen.

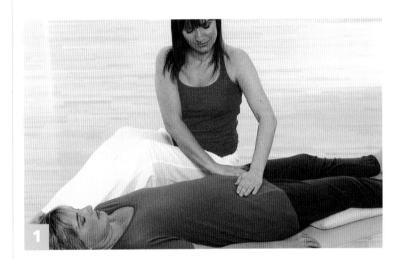

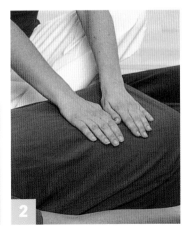

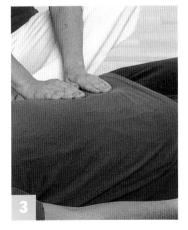

Sex Drive & Stress

This treatment stimulates the adrenal glands, which regulate stress response, metabolism and sex drive. It could therefore be used to help to reduce stress levels, to address weight issues or to give your libido a boost.

1 Place your hands one hand-width lower than Back Position 2 (see p. 16), so that the base of one palm is touching the fingertips of the other one.

2 Use Back Position 3 (see p. 16), placing your hands on the lower ribs, above the kidneys.

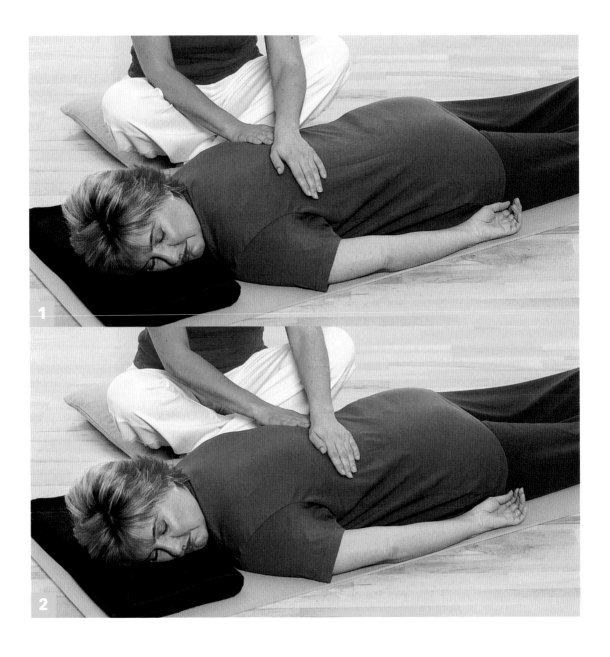

Metabolism & Weight Problems

The following treatment is beneficial for the thyroid, pineal and pituitary glands, as well as the hypothalamus. It balances the metabolism and is useful when you are experiencing weight problems, whether you are over- or underweight.

1 Place one hand directly over the thyroid on the front of the throat and lay the other on the centre of the top of the head.

Suggestion: You can use the same position to treat yourself when you feel your metabolism is working slowly.

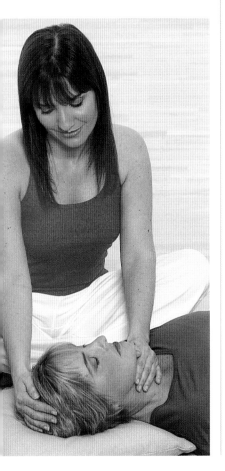

Hot Flushes, Emotional Upsets & Sleeping Problems

The pineal and pituitary glands are connected to the hypothalamus, which controls the release of most hormones by nerve impulse. The following Reiki hand positions balance them, thus helping with emotional disturbances, sleeping irregularities and problems with the body's temperature.

1 Use Head Position 1 (see p. 12), covering the forehead, eyes and cheeks to relax the body.

2 Lay your hands on top of the head horizontally, so that the outer edge of the lower hand touches the curve of the back of the head.

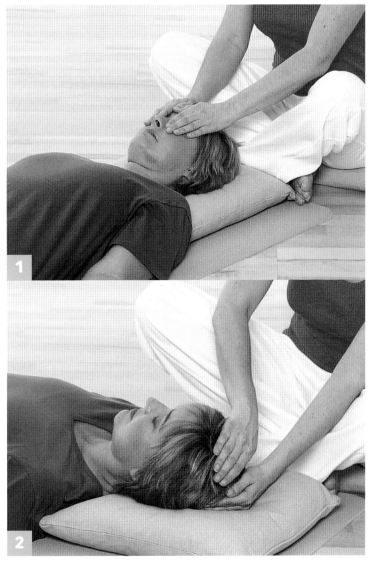

Midlife crisis

The so-called "midlife crisis" is a challenging life stage that we all have to face to varying degrees. It can start any time around the age of forty or fifty, when we become aware that half of our time on earth may have passed and, therefore, we start looking back on our life, reassessing the way we have been living. This transition gives us the opportunity to change our perspective. We become more interested in being as authentic as possible and in deciding how we can use our remaining time and energy in life to do what we really always wanted to do.

The middle years are definitely a turning point. Encountering this phase in a conscious and honest way will enable us to find our own strength, a new identity and heightened self-awareness. If we are open and willing to honour our own life's wisdom, we will discover new, exciting possibilities that will make life interesting and all the more worth living.

People in their middle years are looking for new methods that inspire them to shape their lives into something more nourishing. Many people, therefore, become interested in alternative therapies, such as Reiki, as they acknowledge that it is worth investing in themselves.

Reiki can help by making the strength and trust available to us that we need to make changes in life. The Mental Healing technique – taught in the Second Degree – is useful during this period to ask for inner guidance (see p. 24).

Sense of Well-being: Self-treatment

If you wake early in the morning feeling unsettled, immediately treat yourself with Reiki to improve your mood and outlook on the day. These positions are also helpful when you experience disturbances in your usual sleeping patterns. Additionally, they stimulate your digestion. Maintain each hand position for about five minutes.

1 Place your hands on your pubic bone, using Front Position 4 (see p. 20).

2 Place your hands on the area of your lower ribcage, using Front Position 2 (see p. 20).

3 Continue treating your heart, using Front Position 1 (see p. 20).

4 Lay your hands on the back of the head, using Head Position 4 (see p. 19).

5 Lay your hands over the face, fingers close together, covering your forehead and eyes, using Head Position 1 (see p. 18).

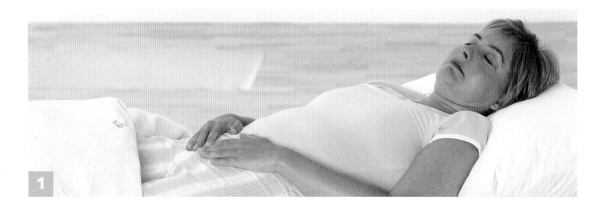

1

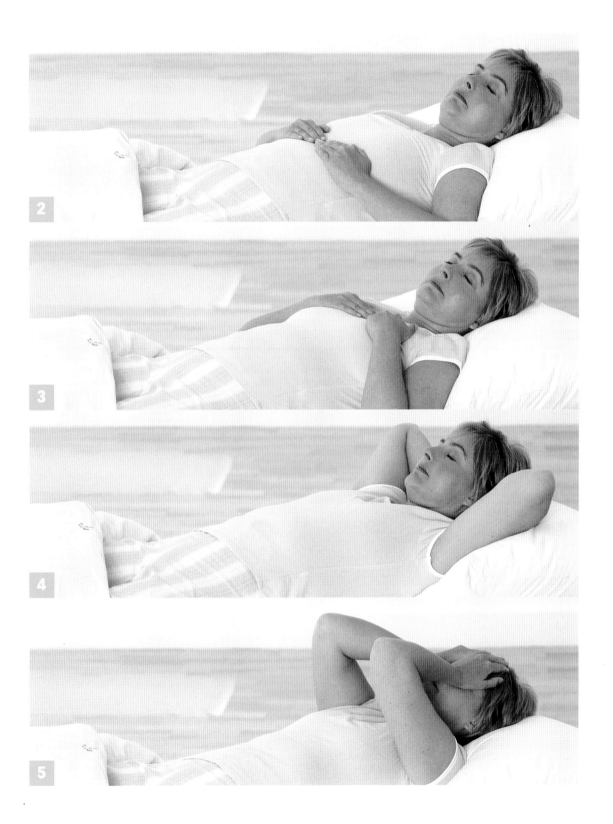

Dealing with Insomnia: Self-treatment

In midlife and during the onset of the menopause, our sleeping patterns often alter. Whenever we wake up in the early morning hours and are unable to get back to sleep, we can use the opportunity to refresh the body and mind with Reiki. This simple technique has quite a strong effect on the mind and the nervous system.

This exercise includes watching your breath while giving Reiki, which takes the attention away from your overly active mind. You simply "watch" your breath coming in and going out, keeping your hands in each position for about five minutes.

1 As soon as you become aware of coming out of sleep, place your hands on your lower belly and give Reiki here.

2 Keeping your hands here, allow yourself to become aware of the rise and fall of the belly. Start observing your breath going in and out. To help keep your attention on your breath, you can silently say the word "in" when breathing in and "out" when breathing out.

3 Now place your hands over your solar plexus, on the right and left sides of your lower ribs, with fingertips touching in the middle. Allow Reiki energy to flow into this area and continue to pay attention to your breathing, still saying "in" and "out" on the breath to help you focus.

4 Rest both hands on the chest and allow Reiki to flow into this area. Notice any sensations in your hands and continue to observe your breathing.

5 Lay one hand on your forehead and the other below the navel. This position will relax you deeply. While giving Reiki to this area, continue to focus on your breath and become aware of any sensations occurring in your body.

Suggestion: This exercise can also be used to refresh and recharge your batteries first thing in the morning. If you have difficulties getting to sleep at night in the first place, however, it is best to do the Reiki treatment shown on page 94: *Reiki Before Sleep.*

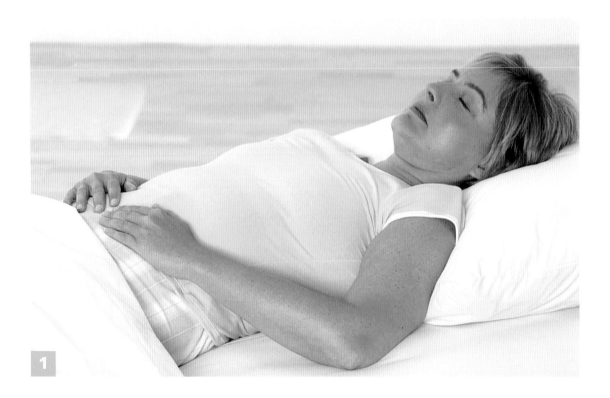

1

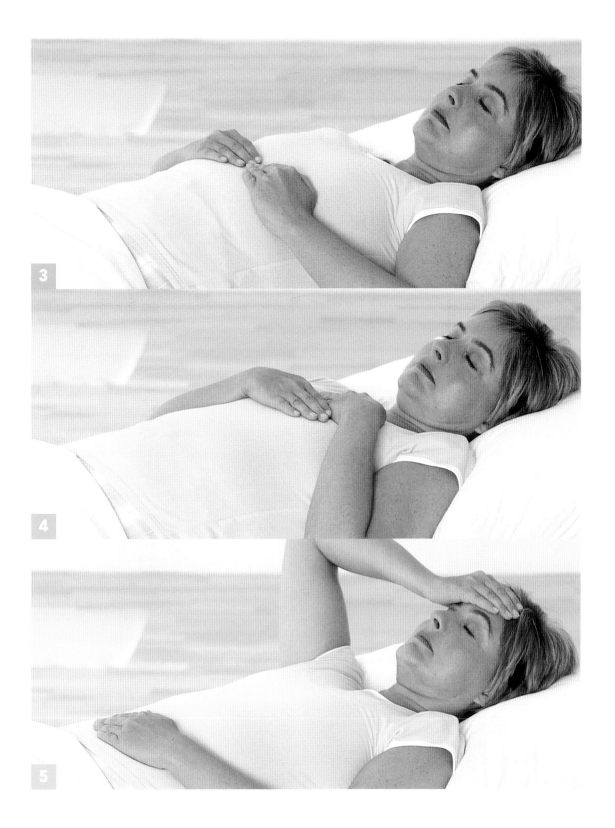

Empty-nest syndrome

THE EMPTY-NEST SYNDROME is a name for what some parents experience when their grown-up children finally leave home. They find it difficult to let go of the "children" and feel there is now a gap in their life. Such parents often feel that they have been so busy devoting all of their time and energy to their children that they have lost part of their own identity and no longer see themselves as separate, independent entities with their own desires and needs. Women, in particular, have often come to equate their sense of self-worth with being needed and, as such, the challenge is to realise that they themselves are important.

It is helpful for parents to try to see the change as an opportunity to release their grip on whatever they perceive they are losing and begin to uncover a new direction in life. A couple's focus has to move back to themselves and their own relationship. They might need, for example, to find new ways of relating to their partner and even new things to do together now that they have all this time with each other again – and this can be difficult. It is good to remember, however, that all our experiences simply show us how to live more fully and authentically.

Reiki can help you to stay grounded and at ease with yourself through this difficult phase. It is good to give yourself or ask someone else to give you daily treatments if possible (see pp. 12–21). The *Menopause* treatments are also very useful during this time (see pp. 126–9).

Balancing your Chakras: Self-treatment

The balancing of the energy centres, or chakras, with Reiki is an extremely effective way of making you feel nourished, peaceful and harmonised. It supports your energy to flow more freely and keeps you happier and healthier. Leave your hands in each position for about five minutes, which makes a total treatment time of approximately twenty-five minutes. You can also play gentle, relaxing music in the background if you wish.

1 Sit on a chair or lie comfortably on your back, close your eyes and relax. Breathe deeply a few times, and while breathing out, allow your body to sink deeper into the surface beneath you.

2 Place your left hand on your forehead, covering your sixth chakra, the space between your eyebrows, and the right hand over your pubic bone, where your first chakra, or root chakra, is located. This balances the energy of your head and the lower parts of your body and brings you more in touch with your sexual energy.

3 Lay your left hand over your throat and your right hand on your belly, below the navel. This balances the energy in your fifth and second chakras, enabling you to feel more connected with your emotions and desires. It also helps you to be able to express and communicate them more easily, and you will feel revitalised and energised.

4 Lay your left hand on the middle of your chest, where your fourth chakra (heart chakra) is located, and the other hand on the solar plexus (third chakra). The heart represents love and compassion and the solar plexus your own strength and power. When these centres are balanced, you will make the right decisions from a place of love and understanding.

5 Place your left hand on your belly where the second chakra is located and your right hand over the forehead, where your sixth chakra is. This position will relax you deeply and help you to let go of all thoughts and feelings. Allow a feeling of peace to spread from this place into the whole body.

6 Now let go of both hands and place them at your sides. Take a couple of moments to enjoy this and then, if you feel like it, wiggle your fingers and toes and stretch your body gently before slowly returning to normal consciousness.

The Chakras

 Crown chakra (seventh)

 Third eye chakra (sixth)

 Throat chakra (fifth)

 Heart chakra (fourth)

 Solar plexus chakra (third)

 Sacral chakra (second)

 Root chakra (first)

"I use Reiki to balance my own energies and nourish myself. It helps me on my spiritual journey."

ANGELA, 48, REIKI STUDENT

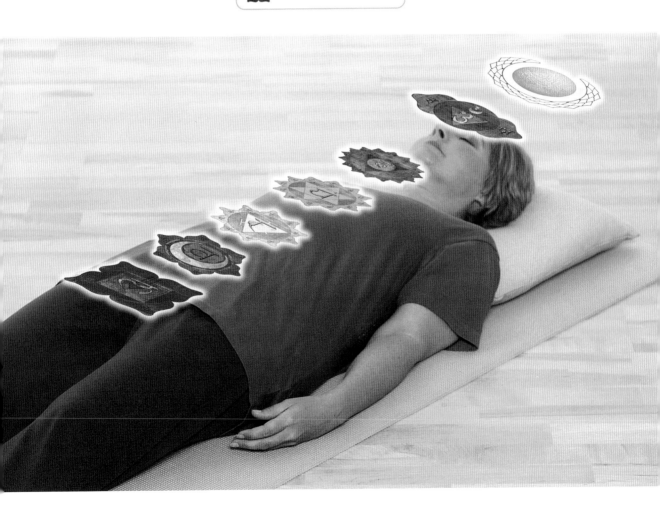

Bereavement

WHEN SOMEONE DIES WHO IS VERY CLOSE TO US, such as our beloved partner or child, we can be in a state of shock for weeks and months afterwards. Although we might feel sad, the full awareness and finality of the loss has probably not yet been fully realised. The emotional pain of the loss seems to be so unbearable that we subconsciously try to numb ourselves from it – out of fear of losing control of our life and going crazy with grief.

Many of us have a deep fear of grief. We experience it as being hopeless and helpless, and we often resist grieving because we don't trust that we can come out the other side of the dark tunnel. However, it is important not to avoid feeling the pain when you lose someone close to you. After having dealt with all the practicalities and arrangements, it is crucial that you give yourself some time to encounter your innermost emotional reactions to the event.

You might face a variety of feelings in the beginning, from anger and resentment at being left behind, or frustration and helplessness at not being able to change the situation, to deep sadness, guilt, pain and grief. If we insist instead on keeping busy, we will close our hearts and simply substitute one pain for another.

We all need to learn to transform our own suffering and, in this way, prepare spiritually for our own death, as well as for the death of friends and family around us. For example, if we discover that we have a life-threatening disease of some description, we need to learn to understand and potentially to let go of the situation. This process involves repeatedly facing grief as we move into ever-deeper levels of realisation. Each time we do this will

be another step towards being able to accept fully our illness and – eventually – accept death peacefully.

To feel that it is safe to grieve, we need the support of others – compassionate friends and relatives who can listen and bear witness to our suffering, respond to our needs with courage and love, give us hope that we can bear the pain, and allow us to feel safe in expressing our sorrow. No matter what our circumstances are, we need to feel respected and unconditionally accepted.

Reiki can be used to support family and friends through their grieving process. It can help them to let go fully, with love, and the physical contact can help to comfort them, as a loving, heart-warming hug would. You can also offer yourself a daily Reiki treatment (see pp. 18–21) to help you through times of personal loss and grief. This creates an intimate space within yourself where you can become more able to acknowledge your innermost feelings and eventually let go of them. You will find it particularly useful to spend some extra time in all the Head Positions (see pp. 18–19), Front Positions 1 and 3 (see p. 20) and Back Position 3 (see p. 21).

Illness, loss, death and grief are powerful transitions, but it is important to recognise that they are also opportunities for us to wake up from any self-centred, materialistic or unhealthy patterns that we might have fallen into. Bereavement can be a time of despair and disorientation, but it can also be a time for renewal of one's own life. Reiki can offer a refuge in the midst of our deepest pain and a means of discovering new depths of meaning in life.

OSHO Nadabrahma Meditation: Self-treatment

This meditation, based on an ancient Tibetan technique, has a powerful calming and healing effect, balancing your energies and harmonising the heart centre. In ancient times, Tibetan monks did the Nadabrahma meditation early every morning, but you can do it at any time of the day where you can set aside an hour. Special music has been recorded to help guide you through the stages of this meditation (see p. 144). It can also be done in silence if you do not have the music.

1 Sit in a relaxed position with your eyes and your mouth closed. Make a humming sound for thirty minutes, loud enough so that you can hear yourself. Imagine your body is hollow inside, like a tube, and that it becomes filled with the vibration of your humming. A point will come when the humming continues by itself and you can become the listener. There is no special breathing technique and you can alter the pitch and move your body gently as you hum, if you like.

2 Keeping your eyes closed, hold your hands in front of your navel, palms facing upwards. Then slowly start to move them away from the centre of your body in two large, flat circles to your sides. Keep the movement of the hands and arms very slow and conscious for 7½ minutes. Feel that you are giving out energy to the universe.

3 Then turn your palms downwards, and reverse the direction of the circles, so that they are coming back towards the centre of your body for another 7½ minutes. Feel yourself receiving energy.

4 With your eyes still closed, sit or lie down on your back and remain still and silent for fifteen minutes before resuming any normal activity.

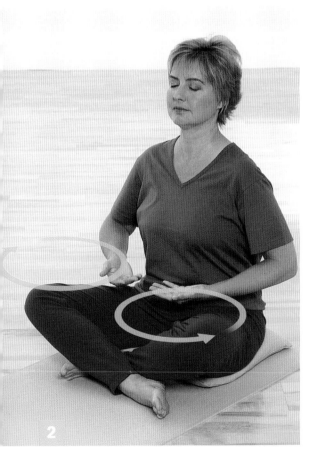

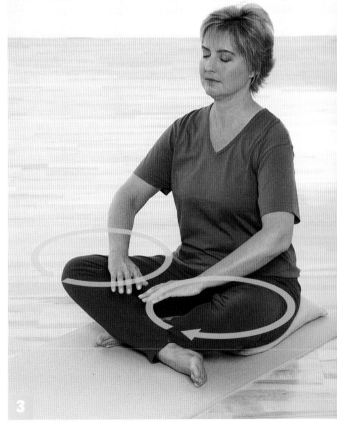

Transition

Transition is a state of existence between one's past and future reality – a time of profound change and uncertainty, since our known world is dissolving and the future, our next existence, has not yet manifested. The moment of death, the end of the physical life form, is the most powerful transition an individual can experience.

We are brought up in a culture that fears death and hides it from us. However, whether we are aware of it or not, death is our constant companion – part of the reality of life. It will come to everyone. Most of the time we try to ignore the fact that we are getting old, getting sick, or losing someone we love. We don't want to see these events as natural occurrences or acknowledge the sands of time slipping through our fingers.

When physical death happens to a friend or relative, we are reminded that we, too, will one day die. Death can come at any time, not just to the sick or elderly. It might happen to us tomorrow. But the enemy is not death; the enemy is our own ignorance and denial. The more we avoid thinking about or preparing for death, the more we are bound to suffer when we – or loved ones – face death. It is important to remember that death is not the end; it is the mere letting go of this physical life form.

On a spiritual plane, death can be viewed as an extraordinary opportunity for the complete liberation and realisation of one's true nature. The body and ordinary mind both die, but another aspect of our being – our innermost essence – continues after death.

As a non-intrusive complementary healing art, Reiki is soothing and comforting to the dying, whether they are at home or in a hospital or hospice. Reiki can give gentle support and make the process of transition much easier for all involved by creating a feeling of acceptance and

"For life and death are one, even as the river and the sea are one."

KAHLIL GIBRAN, *THE PROPHET*, **1923**

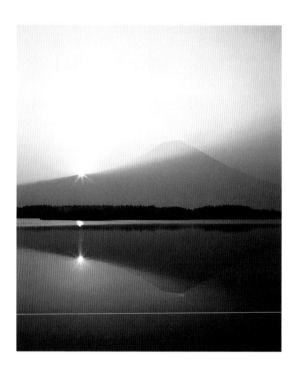

peace. Receiving Reiki helps the person to relax and stay present in the moment of death. The person will feel protected and will find it easier to let go and move into another dimension peacefully. Being present when a person leaves the body is a deeply moving experience – it seems as if they are more aware of themselves and of the inner light within them.

A Tibetan Lama once said: "It is important to give your dying friend or relative all your love, and let him go. Tell him not to worry about anything and let him die in peace, feeling loved."

Helping a Dying Friend

Reiki is a subtle and powerful method that helps and supports the journey of a dying person. It works on all levels – physical, emotional, mental and spiritual – and can, therefore, heal old wounds and bring harmony for family members and loved ones, as well as for the dying person.

1 Give Reiki to the parts of the receiver's body that are most uncomfortable or painful.

2 Treat the middle of the chest so that the heart can let go of this life and welcome transition.

3 Use the Head Positions (see pp. 12–13) to encourage the receiver to feel secure and to let go peacefully.

4 Hold their hand to remind them that they are loved and cherished.

5 Hold your hands over the receiver's legs, knees and feet. People close to death are said to hold a lot of energy and fear in their knees. Receiving Reiki here helps them to let go and trust.

6 Also feel free to give a full Reiki treatment (see pp. 12–17), especially in the days before the final transition happens. If the person is ill, you will release some of the pain.

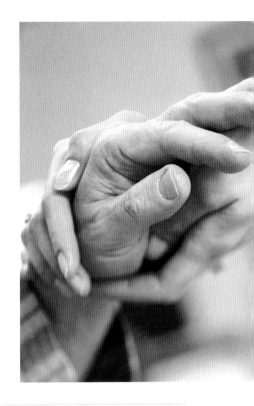

Distant Healing

We can use Reiki Distant Healing to transfer healing energy over long distances when it is physically impossible for us to be with a dying friend or loved one. It is also a good way to offer our final goodbye.

1 Sit in a quiet room, close your eyes and centre yourself by silently giving Reiki to your eyes.

2 Visualise the ill or dying person in your head and get a clear picture of the room where the person is. Second Degree practitioners, raise your hands in front of you and draw the First Reiki symbol in the air to help the process.

3 Keeping your hands raised, Second Degree practitioners draw the Third Reiki symbol over an enlarged visualisation of the receiver's forehead, and then the First Reiki symbol on top.

4 Keeping your hands raised, Second Degree practitioners visualise the symbols in golden light, and say their mantras three times. Then, say the person's name three times.

5 Next, say: "*I am sending you this healing energy in love. You can use it now or any time that is appropriate for you.*"

6 Now hold your hands on either side of the visualised receiver's head (now normal size again) for a few minutes.

7 Second Degree practitioners draw the First Reiki symbol on the chest of the visualised receiver and keep your hands there for three minutes. Then do the same on the visualisation of their stomach, upper back and lower back.

Suggestion: You can talk to your dying loved one from a higher consciousness by drawing the Second Reiki symbol between you and the visualised person and saying your final goodbye.

Reiki beginners can follow the same process, but simply hold your hands either in the air in front of you or on the specified body area instead of drawing the symbols and uttering the mantras.

Chakras

Each of the body's energy centres, known as chakras, relates to different qualities, and the varying Reiki hand positions allow you to tap into these valuable attributes:

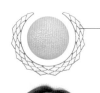

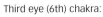

Crown (7th) chakra:
Creates wisdom, intuition, spiritual awareness and oneness.

Third eye (6th) chakra:
Strengthens understanding, inspiration and meditation.

Throat (5th) chakra:
Supports self-expression, creativity, communication and a sense of responsibility.

Heart (4th) chakra:
Increases love, peace, trust, compassion and spiritual development.

Solar plexus (3rd) chakra:
Provides power, determination and strength.

Sacral (2nd) chakra:
Enhances self-esteem, the enjoyment of life, sensuality and sex drive.

Root (1st) chakra:
Strengthens the will to live, enhances fertility and provides a sense of grounding.

Glossary

Affirmation A phrase or word describing a positive condition that we wish for ourselves.

Attunements Special initiations in Reiki energy, also known as energy transmissions. These open a channel for the healing energies in the chakras.

Aura The energy field surrounding the body; a subtle, invisible essence. The human aura can be rendered visible by Kirlian photography. The innermost etheric and emotional bodies are the easiest to discern.

Chakra Circular energy centres in the human subtle body. There are seven main chakras and they are located in the etheric body (see also left). The word *chakra* comes from the Sanskrit, meaning "wheel". On the physical plane, the chakras coincide approximately with the endocrine system in the body.

Channel A person whose inner healing channel has been opened to the subtle energies of Reiki, so that they can flow through that person and be used for healing others or for self-healing.

Chiropractic A healing technique that is based on the theory that disease and disorders are caused by a misalignment of the bones, especially of those in the spine, and that these misalignments prevent the proper functioning of the nerves.

Distant Healing A form of Reiki healing that allows you to send healing energies to a person or situation not in your physical presence.

Emotional body The part of the body's energy field that lies between the etheric and mental bodies. It is related to our emotional state, the part of ourselves thought to be capable of separating from the physical body, as in dreaming or out-of-body experiences.

Endorphins The body's "happiness hormones". These chemicals, known as neurotransmitters, are produced in the brain before being distributed to the rest of the body via the bloodstream, and are thought to help to combat stress.

Energy transmission *see* Attunements.

Etheric body The energetic counterpart of the physical body in which the chakras are located.

Forehead chakra Also popularly known as the Third Eye, this chakra is responsible for clairvoyance, telepathy and spiritual awakening. It is stimulated by meditation.

Hara The Japanese word for the sacral chakra, which, in Eastern tradition, is the best known of the energy centres.

Higher Self The part of us that is divine. We receive guidance from it in, for example, Mental Healing.

Hypothalamus Centrally located on the underside of the brain, the hypothalamus controls involuntary functions, such as maintaining body temperature, as well as the release of hormones into the bloodstream.

Kirlian photography A special technique allowing the aura to become visible through photography. Developed in 1961 by Semyon Davidovitch Kirlian and Valentina Kirliana.

Lymphatic system A system of narrow tubes, called lymph vessels, running throughout the body. Lymph is a clear fluid that circulates around all body tissues. The lymphatic system helps to maintain the correct balance of fluids in the blood and tissues, as well as removing cellular waste products and bacteria in order to help the body fight disease.

Mantra Words and sounds that set subtle energies in vibration; these are used in meditations and in Reiki energy transmissions.

Meditation A still state of not thinking, not wanting, not doing – the ultimate state of relaxation.

Mental Healing Healing through the mind by the emission of gathered mental energy. It can also take place in the form of Distant Healing.

Meridians Energy lines running through the entire body that transport life energy to the organs; by stimulating a meridian we balance and activate the function of each organ.

Sacrum The bony plate situated above the cleft of the buttocks.

Sanskrit An ancient Indian language and the foundation of many modern languages. Hindi sacred texts are written in Sanskrit.

Solar plexus Part of the body that is the seat of the expression of power and emotional control. It is the power wisdom centre of the body.

Subtle body The part of the body that is invisible to normal sight and is charged with higher vibration – a layered energy field permeating and enveloping the physical body. It is thought to be composed of increasingly refined frequencies. The different bands of frequencies form the subtle bodies, each with differing properties, and all of which are essential for the development of a complete person.

Sufism A group of seekers and mystics who originally came from Islam.

Superconscious mind A level within us that is conscious and full of light. The superconscious mind corresponds with the Higher Self, which both knows and sees things clearly. Also known as intuition or spiritual guidance.

Symbol A Symbol comprises a pictorial representation and a name, or mantra. The Reiki Symbols work on the body's healing channel, causing it to vibrate, and so increasing the vibrational frequency of the entire body.

Third eye *see* Forehead chakra.

Thymus gland A gland of the endocrine system, which, when activated, positively stimulates the human immune system.

Universal Life Force The basic energy comprising the whole manifest Universe and lying behind everything we are aware of. When it animates a living organism, the Universal Life Force becomes the life force.

Index

Acknowledgements

Author's Acknowledgements

I want to thank Peter Campbell and Carol Neiman for reading the manuscript and giving me feedback. Thanks also to Jo Godfrey Wood and Kelly Thompson, who edited the English text. Many thanks to my Reiki students, who have shared their experiences with me and made the book so much richer. And finally, thanks to the Osho International Foundation, Switzerland (www.osho.com), for allowing us to use Osho meditation techniques in this book.

Publisher's Acknowledgements

Gaia Books would like to thank the following people for their help with the production of this book: Jonathan Hilton for editorial assistance and Kathie Gill for indexing; Michelle Grant, Juliette Meeus, Leela Itzler, Laura Campbell, Megan Campbell, Martha Schermuly, Nick Hopper and, of course, Monty the dog for modelling; Arthur Barham for photographic assistance; Roisin Donaghy and Lisa Coleman for make-up.

Photographic Acknowledgements

Special photography © Octopus Publishing Group Limited/Mike Good.
All other photography: Banana Stock 57; Corbis/Jon Feingersh 139; Ingram Publishing 9, 11; Octopus Publishing Group Limited/Ruth Jenkinson 41; Photodisc 23, 39, 63, 80-81, 97, 121, 122, 123.

Recommended Reading:

A Gaia Busy Person's Guide to Reiki: Simple routines for home, work & travel, Tanmaya Honervogt & Carol Neiman, Gaia Books (2005)

Meditation: The First and Last Freedom, Osho, St. Martin's Griffin (2004)

Inner Reiki – A practical guide for healing and meditation, Tanmaya Honervogt, Gaia Books (2001)

Reiki – Healing and harmony through the hands, Tanmaya Honervogt, Gaia Books (1998)

Recommended Music & Guided CDs

Tanmaya has created a range of CDs for guided Reiki healing and meditation:

Heal yourself with Reiki – 18 Stages for Self-healing.

Inner Healing, with music by Deva Premal & Miten – for *Eleven Stages of Inner Healing* – with Gayatri Mantra (see pp. 84–5).

Reiki Wellbeing, with music by Georg Deuter – for *Enhanced Wellbeing* (see p. 93) and *Reiki Before Sleep* (see p. 94).

Tanmaya also recommends:
Osho Nadabrahma Meditation CD, New Earth Records, for *Osho Nadabrahma Meditation for Couples* (see p. 44) and *Osho Nadabrahma Meditation* (see p. 137).

For further details of reading material, music and guided healings, visit: www. tanmaya.info.